A COMMUNITY REINFORCEMENT APPROACH TO ADDICTION TREATMENT

The community reinforcement approach (CRA) to treating alcohol and other drug problems is designed to make changes in the client's daily environment, to reduce substance abuse and promote a healthier lifestyle. It is of proven effectiveness, and should be more widely used. This is the first book to present research on the effectiveness of the CRA for a clinical readership. It includes the original study comparing CRA with traditional treatments of alcohol dependence, and summarizes other trials with alcohol, cocaine and heroin users.

The CRA program provides basic guidelines for clinicians, focussing on communication skills, problem solving and drink-refusal strategies, and addresses the needs of the client as part of a social community. Combining practical advice on such matters with a scientific survey of CRA in use, this book offers a new treatment approach to all involved with the support and treatment of those with alcohol and drug problems.

ROBERT J. MEYERS is Research Lecturer in the Department of Psychology and Senior Research Scientist in the Center on Alcoholism, Substance Abuse and Addictions, University of New Mexico. An internationally known researcher and lecturer, he has been involved in the research and treatment of alcohol problems for more than 25 years, and is one of the original collaborators in the first outpatient trial of the Community Reinforcement Approach.

WILLIAM R. MILLER is Distinguished Professor of Psychology and Psychiatry, University of New Mexico. He has many previous publications on the treatment of alcohol problems and other addictive behaviors, and has designed treatment approaches and assessment tools for the addiction field.

INTERNATIONAL RESEARCH MONOGRAPHS IN THE ADDICTIONS (IRMA)

Series Editor
Professor Griffith Edwards
National Addiction Centre
Institute of Psychiatry, London

A series of volumes presenting important research from major centers around the world on the basic sciences, both biological and behavioral, that have a bearing on the addictions, and also addressing the clinical and public health applications of such research. The series will cover alcohol, illicit drugs, psychotropics and tobacco, and is an important resource for clinicians, researchers and policy-makers.

Also in this series:

Cannabis and Cognitive Functioning
Nadia Solowij
ISBN 0 521 159114 7

Alcohol and the Community: A Systems Approach to Prevention
Harold D. Holder
ISBN 0 521 59187 2

A COMMUNITY REINFORCEMENT APPROACH TO ADDICTION TREATMENT

Edited by

ROBERT J. MEYERS and WILLIAM R. MILLER

Psychology Department and the Center on Alcoholism,
Substance Abuse and Addictions,
University of New Mexico

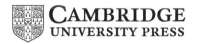
CAMBRIDGE
UNIVERSITY PRESS

CAMBRIDGE UNIVERSITY PRESS
Cambridge, New York, Melbourne, Madrid, Cape Town, Singapore, São Paulo

Cambridge University Press
The Edinburgh Building, Cambridge CB2 2RU, UK

Published in the United States of America by Cambridge University Press, New York

www.cambridge.org
Information on this title: www.cambridge.org/9780521771078

First published 2001
This digitally printed first paperback version 2006

A catalogue record for this publication is available from the British Library

Library of Congress Cataloguing in Publication data

A community reinforcement approach to addiction treatment/edited by Robert J. Meyers,
William R. Miller.
    p.   cm. – (International research monographs in the addictions)
Includes bibliographical references and index.
ISBN 0 521 77107 2
1. Substance abuse – Treatment – Social aspects.   2. Community mental health services.
3. Addicts – Rehabilitation.   4. Addicts – Mental health services.   I. Meyers, Robert J.
II. Miller, William R.   III. Series.
[DNLM: 1. Substance-Related Disorders – rehabilitation.   2. Substance-Related
Disorders – therapy.   3. Community Health Services.   4. Reinforcement (Psychology).
5. Socioenvironmental Therapy. WM 270 C7348 2001]
RC564.C65135 2001
616.86′06–dc21   00-046747

ISBN-13 978-0-521-77107-8 hardback
ISBN-10 0-521-77107-2 hardback

ISBN-13 978-0-521-02634-5 paperback
ISBN-10 0-521-02634-2 paperback

I would like to thank Raphael Pollock, MD, Ph.D., the surgery team, Paula Respondek, PA, and the entire staff at the Sarcoma Unit of The M.D. Anderson Cancer Center who made it possible for me to complete this book. I also want to thank all my family, friends, and colleagues who supported me through this very difficult time. I especially want to thank Marta and Mike Dougher, my good friend and comrade Marcello Maviglia, my brother Charles Meyers, and most of all my best friend and companion Jane Ellen Smith.

R.J.M.

To George Hunt and Nathan Azrin, the founding fathers.

W.R.M.

Contents

Contributors

Patrick J. Abbot
University of New Mexico,
Center on Alcoholism, Substance
Abuse and Addictions,
2350 Alamo SE,
Albuquerque, NM 87106,
USA
e-mail: pabbot@unm.edu

Harold D. Delaney
University of New Mexico,
Psychology Department,
Logan Hall,
Albuquerque, NM 87131,
USA
e-mail: hdelaney@unm.edu

Mark D. Godley
Chestnut Health Systems,
720 West Chestnut,
Bloomington, IL 61701,
USA
e-mail: mgodley@chestnut.org

Kathryn A. Grant
University of New Mexico,
Center on Alcoholism, Substance
Abuse and Addictions,
2350 Alamo SE,
Albuquerque, NM 87106,
USA

Stephen T. Higgins
University of Vermont,
Ira Allen School,
38 Fletcher Place,
Burlington, VT 05401-1419,
USA
e-mail: stephen.higgins@uvm.edu

Robert J. Meyers
University of New Mexico,
Center on Alcoholism, Substance
Abuse and Addictions,
2650 Yale SE,
Albuquerque, NM 87106,
USA
e-mail: bmeyers@unm.edu

Erica J. Miller
University of New Mexico,
Center on Alcoholism, Substance
Abuse and Addictions,
2350 Alamo SE,
Albuquerque, NM 87106,
USA

William R. Miller
University of New Mexico,
Center on Alcoholism, Substance
Abuse and Addictions,
2350 Alamo SE,
Albuquerque, NM 87106,
USA
e-mail: wrmiller@unm.edu

Jane Ellen Smith
University of New Mexico,
Psychology Department,
Logan Hall,
Albuquerque, NM 87131,
USA
e-mail: janellen@unm.edu

J. Scott Tonigan
University of New Mexico,
Center on Alcoholism, Substance
Abuse and Addictions,
2350 Alamo SE,
Albuquerque, NM 87106,
USA
e-mail: jtonigan@unm.edu

Preface

The Community Reinforcement Approach (CRA), as originally applied to the treatment of alcohol problems and as later widened in its application to other substances, has always seemed to have common sense to recommend it. We only need a nodding experience with the behavior of children or a modicum of personal insight to find persuasive evidence that reward can alter behavior patterns. So, make stopping drinking tangibly rewarding, and troubled drinkers may be able to stop drinking – a psychological postulate much in accord with common sense and ordinary life.

In fact, in the treatment world, CRA has enjoyed a rather odd status up to now. Most researchers believe that the evidence for its efficacy is strong and reviewers have repeatedly rated this treatment approach as being better supported by controlled assessments than a galaxy of more widely favored practices. CRA seems to have become a succès d'estime only to be left on the shelf.

This immensely authoritative and comprehensive account of the origins of the CRA concept and the research evidence for its therapeutic benefits must surely do much to counter that previous neglect. It is a book which one must hope to see widely read by clinicians and those responsible for the development and provision of services. Researchers will find in its pages stimulating ideas for new applications and testings.

What is also interesting about this book is that beyond its reporting of the research output it raises questions about how research in this kind of field comes to be made – there is a story here within the story. Research on CRA has been carried forward by a relatively small group of people, most of whom have known each other well, and with ideas and traditions fostered within the group and transmitted across a generation of researchers. It is the continuity in the evolution, the incremental nature of the endeavor, the long slog and the idea followed through which form the deeper story. We need better and more widely to understand how science is made, but meanwhile CRA can provide a case study illustrative of that theme.

The rules for IRMA publications require that all material that has not previously been through peer review will go through external peer review before being accepted, while material which has been previously published in journal form will be scrupulously gone through within the office. We aim at a process which will produce a coherent book rather than at bits put together within covers. The preparation of these monographs is therefore an active process with many demands made on the authors. I am grateful to Robert J. Meyers and William R. Miller and their cast of authors for their courtesy and patience, and believe that the outcome is a statement of landmark significance for its field.

Griffith Edwards
Series Editor

Acknowledgments

The authors and editors would like to acknowledge the support of the National Institute on Alcohol Abuse and Alcoholism and the National Institute on Drug Abuse. Without their assistance these projects would not have been possible.

1

Developing the Community Reinforcement Approach

ROBERT J. MEYERS AND MARK D. GODLEY

The story of the Community Reinforcement Approach (CRA) begins 30 years ago, when indigent alcohol-dependent individuals in downstate Illinois were routinely admitted to the nearest state mental hospital. For the 27 southernmost counties in Illinois, this institution was Anna State Hospital. Despite the fact that nonmedical detoxification programs were established at the Addiction Research Foundation in Ontario, Canada and other locations in the United States, such programs did not become available in rural Illinois until 1975. So in the early 1970s alcohol-dependent individuals were typically placed on the same ward as the general psychiatric population. Thus, it was not uncommon for them to share a ward with patients suffering from acute psychoses, schizophrenia, bipolar disorder, and severe depression. Not surprisingly, many newly admitted alcohol-dependent patients were frightened and confused upon sobering up and finding themselves in such a place. Fortunately, the majority of them adjusted with time over the course of relatively long stays, and some even developed a sense of humor about it. We remember one recovering alcoholic, years later, showing us a postcard of the state hospital that he had sent to a friend. The inscription read, "Having a great time, wish you were here."

Although at the time it was not a common practice, some state hospitals did have special programs for substance abusers. At Anna State Hospital, alcohol-dependent clients slept on the psychiatric ward but during the day they went to the Alcohol Treatment Program (ATP) in a separate building. Here they spent their hours participating in alcohol education classes, and group and individual therapy. Treatment was based on a disease model and the 12 steps of Alcoholics Anonymous. The unit administrator was a social worker, and most of the staff were stable, caring recovering alcoholics. It was in this ATP unit at Anna State Hospital that CRA was born.

CRA was the brain child of George Hunt, a doctoral student in the Department of Educational Psychology at Southern Illinois University in Carbondale. Hunt also worked as a Research Associate in the Behavior Research Laboratory of Dr Nathan Azrin at Anna State Hospital, which is nestled in the Shawnee National Forest 20 miles south of the city. The 1970s were an incredibly productive time for the Azrin group. Under Azrin's direction the research staff of the Behavior Research Laboratory validated and published reports of behavioral interventions for a variety of nervous habits, marital problems, and unemployment, and developed a host of life and social skills training procedures for the developmentally disabled. Some of these treatments were widely circulated through the popular press (e.g., Azrin & Fox, 1976; *Toilet training in less than a day*).

As inpatient treatment began to lose popularity, outpatient therapy became the logical place to experiment with CRA. In August of 1975, Mark Godley accepted the position of Coordinator of Alcohol Treatment Programs at the Mental Health Services of Franklin and Williamson Counties. This was a community mental health center that operated a halfway house and an outpatient program for individuals suffering from alcohol problems. Godley, a social worker, began a 5-year collaboration with Nathan Azrin when he contacted him in the September of that year, about working together on behavioral alcoholism treatment research. Initially it was George Hunt who trained Mark Godley and his one outreach worker. Hunt, a counterculture icon who did not fit the typical research scientist profile, was killed in a sailing accident in the Gulf of Mexico. This left Nathan Azrin and his colleagues to carry on CRA research, which soon led them to the first outpatient CRA trial.

Mark Godley continued his association with Azrin through John Mallams, another doctoral student and Research Associate from Azrin's lab. Mallams had served as a therapist in the second CRA inpatient trial (Azrin, 1976) and was especially eager to work in a community outpatient setting. After Hunt's untimely death, John Mallams became the coordinator of Azrin's alcohol treatment project. Godley and Mallams were both Texans, and that was about all they needed to forge a friendship. Together they decided to carry out a community-based CRA experiment under Azrin's leadership.

In these pioneering days of community-based outpatient services, enthusiasm for a community-based study was high. However, most alcohol programs still adhered to the 12-step approach with cult-like fervor. The local recovering community, like many, regarded any other approach as heretical. This made it extremely difficult to introduce changes in treatment regimens, much less conduct behavioral research on alcohol treatment. Another significant event was the emergence of reports that alcoholics might be able to control their drinking if support was found [(Davies, 1962; Heather & Robertson, 1962; Lovibond and Caddy, 1970), the Rand Report (Armour, Polich, & Stanbul, 1976), and work at the Patton State Hospital (Sobell & Sobell, 1973*a, b*)]. The Sobells and others encouraged Azrin and Mallams to incorporate such procedures as stimulus control and discrimination training, and to use a controlled drinking goal in the next CRA trial. Godley was familiar with and not unsympathetic to these reports, but he was already struggling to gain acceptance as a young, nonrecovering professional in a field dominated by older recovering alcoholics who were singularly interested in Alcoholics Anonymous. Godley had much negotiating to do even to establish a community-based research study of outpatient alcoholics. In the end he was supported by his administrator, Floyd Cunningham, but in the process agreed that including controlled drinking in a research study – no matter how well-managed – would be unacceptable to the recovering community. The likely consequence would be protests, formal complaints, and protracted debates that could hinder or kill the project. In a meeting with Azrin and John Mallams to discuss the future of the collaboration, Godley stated that incorporating a controlled drinking goal was unacceptable to the community. So in order to collaborate they needed to drop controlled drinking from the design. Azrin smiled and said, "OK, we'll leave controlled drinking to the Sobells. We'll do the abstinence approach." The subject was never discussed again.

The new year ushered in change. In December of 1976, Godley and Mallams had an unexpected resignation and a resulting open counselor position. They were eager to recruit someone who would learn CRA and become a therapist in the next study. The outgoing staff member had come to know a young social work student who was interning at the ATP, and had urged him to apply for the position. With his bachelor's degree still incomplete, the student was hesitant to apply, but he finally agreed to interview for the position. This newcomer to the small CRA group was Robert J. Meyers. Meyers had heard that Godley was easy-going, but nothing could have prepared him for the onslaught of questions that John Mallams had ready for him. But at the conclusion of the interview, both Godley and Mallams knew they had found their CRA therapist for the largest CRA study yet. Meyers joined the staff, with Mallams as the clinical director and his CRA mentor, and Godley as the center's director.

Meyers' intensive training began the moment he walked through the door on his first day of work. Mallams was determined to make sure that Meyers knew every procedure for every possible situation. In the course of training and preparation for the first outpatient trial, Mallams and Meyers modified the inpatient procedures. It was also during this time that they developed the sobriety sampling technique and much of the disulfiram monitoring program. The project was quite progressive for its time, as pilot subject sessions with therapists were taped and reviewed to ensure that all clinical staff were similar in their use of CRA. Several months later, Azrin introduced a new graduate student to the laboratory. Robert W. Sisson underwent similar training and scrutiny by Mallams and Meyers.

The next significant event was Azrin's sabbatical year. Mallams created a great deal of enthusiasm for an evaluation of the social and recreational component of CRA, known as the United Club (UC). The UC was basically a "dry" social club that had been a component of prior CRA studies. It had operated out of locations where Hunt or Mallams had been able to negotiate free or low-cost space. It took place at weekends at the Carbondale Community Recreation Center. Conveniently located on the "main drag", where there were many student bars, the UC operated every Saturday night for nearly two years. Few laboratory situations could parallel this setting for observing and teaching social skills. Godley, Meyers, and Sisson became convinced that when a single recovered male alcoholic asked a woman to dance and completed the dance, he was well on his way to recovery! The Saturday night potluck drew in 80 to 100 recovering people who assembled to hear live country and western music, play poker for cigarettes, shoot pool, and converse. A randomized trial of the UC found that attendance could be primed through a set of encouragement procedures, and that those encouraged to attend had better outcomes in terms of recovery. The UC study became Mallams' doctoral dissertation and was eventually published in the *Quarterly Journal of Alcohol Studies* (Mallams et al., 1982). Even though many Saturday nights were given up to the UC, looking back we particularly appreciate Mallams' tireless work to keep each night at the UC lively, with the help of just a few dedicated therapists, their supportive spouses, and without any grant funds or user fees. It was during this same year that Meyers and Sisson piloted and shaped the outpatient procedures into their final form.

Azrin had been back from his sabbatical for less than a year when Mallams accepted another position, leaving Meyers and Sisson as the heirs apparent to CRA. During that first year most clients were seen simulta-neously by two therapists, with each taking turns as the lead counselor. At the conclusion of a session, one therapist would debrief the other by discussing each procedure used and whether it appeared to be helpful. In addition to practising therapy in tandem and listening to therapy tapes together, much of Meyers' and Sisson's socializing time was spent discuss-ing and arguing about how CRA should be properly done.

As noted, CRA had only been conducted in an inpatient setting before 1976. Both early trials had been completed at Anna State Hospital, where the clients were severely dependent and held by physician or legal commit-ment. Now it was time to try CRA as an outpatient program. Several years of preparation were required before the 1982 trial could begin. This was a time of great excitement and high energy, but we soon learned that we had been quite naive. Working with outpatient clients presented a new chall-enge: keeping people in treatment. CRA had only been done with a captive audience up to that point. So before the first outpatient CRA trial began, our team treated literally hundreds of clients as practice cases. Most of the cases were audio-taped and then reviewed. Discussions ensued about the proper way to use a procedure, or, more importantly, about which procedure should have been used in the first place. The process was arduous and critical. Revision on the proper use of each procedure some-times took months, and during that time clients were already being intro-duced to the newly revised version. When clients failed to comply with our neatly designed procedures, our group typically concluded that we were not executing the procedures properly. We expected success, and were determined to achieve it. As a result of our work with these less predictable and less compliant outpatients, the CRA procedures multiplied and their order of implementation became more flexible. Importantly, a menu of alternatives from which the therapist could choose emerged. In the course of this process the grave importance of the first few sessions became apparent. Meyers and Sisson came to understand the need to look for ways to "hook" the client into treatment early, to get the client interested and engaged. In retrospect, the term "hooking" seems harsh, and current language focuses more on "motivating". Whatever the process is called, unless clients become motivated, curious, or even excited about the change process, they will never follow through with procedures or stay in treat-ment. Over time Meyers and Sisson developed a positive clinical style that retained the CRA procedures while also building rapport and trust.

Through seeing many clients and reviewing hundreds of hours of tapes, the motivational process became clearer: it involved finding the client's reinforcement. But a debate emerged over which came first: the procedure or the reinforcer. Does the proper procedure elicit the reinforcers, or do we need to find the proper reinforcers first in order to use a procedure? Meyers believed that it was strictly the social and recreational reinforcers that served as the catalyst for change. Sisson thought that compliance procedures for disulfiram maintenance needed to be in place in order to enforce abstinence. Regardless, our early CRA work taught us that therapy needs to focus on how to identify appropriate reinforcers. These reinforcers were then integrated into CRA procedures. Social and recreational reinforcers seemed to be some of the strongest, but often they could not stand alone, at least not at first. Disulfiram could help sometimes, but one needed proper reinforcers to take disulfiram.

With the outpatient CRA trial complete, Meyers left Illinois in 1982 for New Mexico. Between 1982 and 1986 Meyers was the director of several community-based alcohol treatment programs. In 1986 Meyers went to work for the Center on Alcoholism, Substance Abuse, and Addictions (CASAA) at the University of New Mexico, where William Miller was seeking to launch a clinical trial. In 1988 they submitted the first of a series of collaborative projects, and they have been working together on a variety of CRA treatment research studies ever since. As for the original CRA researchers in Southern Illinois, Mark Godley, the last of the original Azrin outpatient group, left Southern Illinois in 1987 for a position at Chestnut Health Systems in Bloomington, Illinois. Around that same time Azrin himself moved to Nova University in Fort Lauderdale.

One of the puzzling and frustrating questions during the two decades of CRA work represented in this book is why this effective treatment method has not been more widely adopted in clinical practice. Researchers must take as much responsibility for this as clinicians. Too often, research findings are published only in scientific journals, and in language relatively inaccessible to practitioners. An important motivation behind the publication of this book and of a therapist guide (Meyers & Smith, 1995) has been to make CRA more comprehensible and accessible to clinicians who treat substance use disorders. At the turn of the century, CRA is the product of 30 years of clinical experience with hundreds of patients. It has been rigorously tested not only by Azrin's group (Chapter 2), but also in the other studies described in detail in this book. To date, every clinical trial has shown that CRA has a better outcome compared with more traditional treatment practices. CRA procedures are now well specified and relatively easy to learn. We puzzle now about the necessary reinforcers for clinicians in order to get them to try this method in their practice.

2

Practice and Promise: The Azrin Studies

ERICA J. MILLER

In the early 1970s, George Hunt and his advisor, Nathan Azrin, developed a theory for describing the etiology and maintenance of alcohol problems and a therapy approach for addressing how to treat them. Based on learning theory, and in particular on the operant approach described by Skinner (1938), their Community Reinforcement Approach (CRA) for the treatment of alcohol dependence stressed the interaction between a person's behavior and the environment. Until this time, most alcohol treatment programs had focused on the treatment of the individual and had greatly ignored the importance of the individual's social environment. Hunt and Azrin proposed that the etiology of alcohol problems was influenced by patterns of positive and negative reinforcement. Specifically, drinking was believed to be maintained by the reinforcing properties of its subjective effects (e.g., pleasant and relaxing feelings), physical sensations (e.g., taste), social rewards, and dependence-inducing qualities. These sources of reinforcement could possibly maintain drinking indefinitely, depending on the accumulated strength of these factors for an individual. However, Hunt and Azrin theorized that those with alcohol problems might be deterred from drinking when use of alcohol interfered with other sources of satisfaction and positive reinforcement in their environment. They predicted that drinking could be reduced if reinforcers for *not* drinking, such as a better interpersonal relationship or satisfying employment, were maximized, frequent, and contingent upon not drinking alcohol. To accomplish this goal, CRA attempted to rearrange these contingencies such that sober behavior was more rewarding than drinking behavior.

The initial report of the implementation of CRA was published in 1973 as a dissertation project designed by Hunt and Azrin (Hunt & Azrin, 1973). Azrin and his colleagues designed a series of subsequent studies, testing the relative effectiveness of specific treatment components in order to refine the approach. CRA was first tested on alcohol-dependent individuals in an inpatient setting, then tailored for use with outpatient populations who might otherwise have required residential treatment. Three early, well-designed studies demonstrated CRA to be more effective than the existing standard treatments for alcohol dependence (Azrin, 1976; Azrin et al., 1982; Hunt & Azrin, 1973). In later years, the procedures were modified and extended to include interventions with other client groups and even with significant others of substance abusers.

1973: The initial test of the Community Reinforcement Approach

The initial CRA study (Hunt & Azrin, 1973) evaluated the effectiveness of the treatment for 16 males admitted to a state hospital in a rural Midwestern region and diagnosed with alcoholism (see Table 2.1). Eight drinkers were selected arbitrarily and matched with eight other alcohol-dependent clients based on employment history, family stability, previous drinking history, age, and education. The standard treatment consisted of about 25 hour-long educational lectures and films on Alcoholics Anonymous and on the nature of behavioral, sexual, and physical problems caused by excessive alcohol use. All patients received the same housing, standard treatment program, and other hospital services. A coin flip decided which member of each pair would receive the additional CRA counseling procedures (CRA group) and which would receive only the standard treatment (control group).

CRA treatment components

As was demonstrated in this trial, CRA was best viewed as a treatment "package", rather than a single treatment approach. The treatment consisted of a family of techniques that could be modified in content and varied in order of presentation, depending on the needs of the individual client. For example, in the initial trial the five married clients were joined by their spouses for marital therapy, while the three single clients received a modified version of the same procedures. Likewise, more time was spent on job-finding procedures for clients lacking steady employment, while this portion of the CRA program was limited or eliminated for successfully employed drinkers. Hunt and Azrin introduced five major CRA treatment components during the 1973 trial: job-finding procedures, behavioral

Table 2.1. *Overview of Azrin and Colleagues' early CRA trials*

Participant characteristics	Year of the study 1973	1976	1982
N	16	18	43
Gender	Males	Males	Males, Females
Population	Inpatients	Inpatients	Outpatients
Diagnosis[a]	Alcohol dependent	Alcohol dependent	Alcohol dependent
Mean age (years)	38.31	(Not reported)	33.9
Mean education (years)	10.6	(Not reported)	11.2
% Married/Cohabiting	63%	39%	5%
% With recent or current employment	63%	(Not reported)	46%
Method of group assignment	Matched	Matched	Randomized
Treatment groups (n)	Hospital services (8) CRA (8)	Hospital services (9) CRA (9)	Traditional (14) Disulfiram assurance (DA) (15) CRA + DA (14)
Counseling hours for CRA groups	50	30	6.4

Follow-up results[b]	1973 Hospital	1973 CRA	1976 Hospital	1976 CRA	1982 Traditional	1982 DA	1982 CRA + DA
% Days drinking	79%	14%**	55%	2%**	55%	26%	3%*
% Days unemployed	62%	5%**	56%	20%**	36%	11%	7%
% Days away from family	36%	16%**	67%	7%**	15%	0%	0%
% Days institutionalized	27%	2%**	45%	0.1%**	1%	0%	0%

[a] Participants in each of the three studies met the current criteria for dependence, yet there was no mention as to the severity (e.g., drinks per week) or chronicity of the drinking problem.

[b] In each trial, clients provided information to their counselors during follow-up visits. When possible, the information was verified by collateral report and other methods (e.g., arrest records). Program staff members blind to the research objectives and client treatment assignment collected similar information.

Reports to counselors and staff were well correlated (Pearson's = 95 for the 1973 and 1976 trials; correlations were not reported for the 1982 trial).

Note:* $p < 0.01$, ** $p < 0.005$.

Table 2.2. *The evolution of CRA treatment components across three early studies*

New treatment components added for each trial

Hunt & Azrin (1973)	Azrin (1976)	Azrin *et al.* (1982)
Job finding	Disulfiram prescription	Motivational counseling
Behavioral marital	Disulfiram compliance	Sobriety sampling
therapy	procedure	Drink refusal
Social/leisure counseling	Problem-solving	Immediate disulfiram
Reinforcer access	Buddy system	administration
counseling	Early warning/mood	Muscle relaxation training
Social Club	monitoring	
Home visits		

marital therapy, social and leisure counseling, a Social Club, and home visits (see Table 2.2).

Job-finding

Just prior to Hunt and Azrin's (1973) initial published description of CRA, Jones and Azrin (1973) reported their findings concerning successful and unsuccessful approaches to obtaining employment. At the time, the popular belief was that the important ingredients in successful job-finding involved looking at Want Ads, dressing properly, and filling out applications well. However, Jones and Azrin noted the lack of experimental evidence suggesting that such an approach would lead to an increased probability of obtaining a job. They hypothesized that although such skills could prove to be helpful, other more powerful factors might account for successful job attainment. Based on the principles of social reinforcement theory, they reasoned that the employment process could be viewed as an informal job-information network in which favors were returned with rewards. Specifically, persons knowledgeable about job openings would share this information with unemployed acquaintances who they believed would return the privilege with rewards, such as friendship or diligent work. As part of their research efforts to explore this possibility, Jones and Azrin (1973) surveyed employed individuals about the factors that led them to their current employment situations. In line with their hypothesis, a surprisingly high two-thirds of respondents reported that friends, relatives, or acquaintances provided the initial job lead. In addition, eventual job placement was more likely if the informant and applicant shared a personal, in comparison to a professional, prior relationship.

Based on the results reported in Jones and Azrin's (1973) study, Hunt and Azrin developed a new approach to job-finding for their unemployed clients. During the first session, clients were told that research has shown that their chances of remaining sober are improved if they have a satisfying job. Clients were still guided in improving basic job-finding skills, such as reading ads and practising for interviews. However, the main emphasis was now on recognizing the importance of social contacts for obtaining initial leads and increasing the likelihood of eventual employment. Clients without jobs were instructed to (1) prepare a résumé, (2) read a pamphlet titled, "How to get the job" (Dreese, 1960), (3) contact their friends and relatives on the phone to inform them of the need for employment and to request job leads, (4) call the major factories and plants in the area, (5) place a "Situations-Wanted" ad in the local papers, (6) rehearse the job interview, and (7) fill out applications for the jobs that were available. If necessary, clients were encouraged to cultivate new social contacts for the purpose of joining their job-information networks. Similar to other CRA procedures, the counselor played an active part by role-playing interviews, modeling phone calls to potential employers, and having clients phone contacts during the therapy session.

Behavioral marital therapy

Hunt and Azrin blended together their operant reinforcement approach with the general approach to marital counseling described by Stuart (1969). The specific techniques in their behavioral marital therapy were designed to accomplish three major goals: (1) provide reinforcement for the drinker to be a functioning marital partner, (2) provide reinforcement for the spouse for maintaining the marital relationship, and (3) make the drinking of alcohol incompatible with the improved marital relationship. Communication training and in-session behavioral rehearsal helped clients and their spouses learn effective, positive techniques for interacting with each other both in and out of the session.

During the first session, the drinker and his wife were asked to fill out the Marriage Adjustment Inventory (Manson & Lerner, 1962) in order to identify 12 potential problem areas in the marriage: money management, family relationships, sex problems, children, social life, attention, neurotic tendencies, immaturity, grooming, ideological difficulties, dominance, and general incompatibility. After reviewing the inventory, partners were each instructed to create a list of specific activities their spouse could perform to make them happy or to help repair an identified problem in the relationship. These lists often included items such as preparing a special meal, taking care of the children, engaging in sexual activities at a certain frequency, or spending a night out together. Counselors asked partners to speak directly to one another and to make specific and positive statements when requesting behaviors they would like the other person to do. The nondrinking spouse was instructed only to provide such pleasantries to the drinker when he was sober, thereby rewarding nondrinking behavior. In this way, sober behavior was positively reinforced, while drinking would lead to the withdrawal of positive reinforcement.

For some spouses involved in a relationship with a problem drinker, positive feelings about the marriage had dwindled due to emotional neglect, lack of positive contact, and possibly alcohol-related violent behavior. The emotional disconnection and feelings of resentment sometimes resulted in resistance toward engaging in the positive activities requested by the drinker. In such instances, the counselor aided the couple in devising a plan to compromise. If one of them *refused* to provide a particular type of positive reinforcement, the solution was the introduction of a *reinforcer sampling* procedure. The counselor asked the resistant client to "just try it for 1 week" then return for the next session to discuss whether it should be continued after that time.

Married clients were joined by their spouses for each counseling session. Those clients who were not in a romantic relationship had similar arrangements with a family member or another person who was close to them. For those clients without an adequate support system, a "synthetic" family was created, often including relatives, an employer, or a minister. The synthetic family consisted of persons who would have a reason to maintain regular contact with the drinker and would expect him to behave in particular ways, such as helping with chores. People were chosen with whom the client wished to maintain a positive relationship. In this way, sobriety could remain a condition for maintaining the positive benefits of the relationships, while drinking behavior would result in the loss of contact with, or withdrawal of positive benefits from, the individuals in the synthetic family.

Social and leisure counseling

Recognizing the importance of environmental contingencies for supporting or preventing drinking, Hunt and Azrin developed procedures to
rearrange the drinker's social environment so that it was supportive of
sobriety. Many drinkers would eventually face the challenge of leaving the
treatment center and returning to environments conducive to drinking. In
addition, many had lost important past relationships due to a rift caused
by their excessive drinking, and their current friendships were limited to a
few individuals with drinking problems of their own. In such cases, clients
needed help to re-establish past relationships or to develop new ones with
nondrinking individuals who would associate with them in nondrinking
environments. Clients were encouraged to schedule social interactions
with nondrinking friends, relatives, and community groups, and to refrain
from spending time with friends who drank alcohol. To help clients
recognize potentially rewarding nondrinking leisure activities, counselors
asked clients to list activities that they had always wanted to do but had
not done. Clients were encouraged to sample engaging in these activities
alone or with nondrinking companions to decide if the new activity was
sufficiently enjoyable to compete with the urge to spend time drinking
alcohol.

   Azrin and his colleagues noted that a significant barrier for drinkers
attempting to develop new social contacts and new leisure interests was a
lack of available resources. For example, problem drinkers were often
faced with monetary difficulties, resulting in an inability to pay for certain
leisure activities. At times the lack of resources involved transportation
problems, particularly if a car was not owned or if a driver's license had
been revoked following a driving whilst intoxicated (DWI) arrest. Furthermore, some individuals who had been problem drinkers for many years
found that the resources they were lacking included social skills, such as
being able to talk about current events and popular activities. To address
these issues, Hunt and Azrin developed and implemented the procedures
of *reinforcer-access counseling* and *activity priming*. To increase clients'
access to potentially rewarding nondrinking activities, counselors took an
active role in providing clients with various resources. For example, counselors arranged for clients to obtain a radio or television in their home or to
subscribe to area newspapers and magazines. Since reading about current
events in the newspaper could allow clients to engage in a wider variety of
conversation topics, access to such things aided the client in realizing the

reinforcing properties of a life not dependent on alcohol. When counselors assisted a client in buying a car, obtaining a driver's license, or having a telephone installed, the client could feel more like a member of general society and would be in a better position to have transportation for a job, for example, or receive phone calls from potential employers.

Although most of these reinforcers are viewed as necessities by many people, problem drinkers seemed to find it difficult to provide them for themselves. At times, the clients could not afford to indulge in such niceties. For some clients, the drinking way of life had extended to the point where they seemed to have "forgotten" how to provide these things for themselves. Clients also may have experienced so many failures and disappointments that they had lost the drive to seek positive rewards for themselves. CRA took these factors into account by having counselors "*prime*" these activities in clients. For example, counselors might have paid the initial costs of installing a phone or bought the client plants for the home. These initial favors given to the clients allowed them to sample the positive reinforcers. After the initial priming the client was expected to care for the plants and pay the monthly phone bills, thereby assuming responsibility in order to continue the presence of the reinforcing object or activity.

Social Club

During the course of the initial CRA trial, a local tavern was transformed into a Social Club on Saturday nights for use by clients and their invited guests. Alcohol was not allowed at the club, and intoxicated individuals were turned away. Instead, clients could enjoy an array of nondrinking activities, such as playing card games, listening to a jukebox or a band, dancing, picnics, bingo games, and movies. The Social Club helped clients rebuild a social life that was incompatible with drinking alcohol. It provided a safe place to practise new social interactions and served as a stepping-stone to prepare clients for their return to the larger society.

Home visits

For the first month after discharge from the hospital, clients were visited once or twice weekly by a counselor. After the first couple of months, visits decreased to twice and then to once a month, in addition to contacts made when clients visited the Social Club. Continued support following a return to the client's natural environment was viewed as particularly important, due to the inevitable reintroduction of trigger situations and the potential for relapse. During the counselors' visits, the clients were reminded of the reinforcers which existed for family, job, and social life participation. Counselors aided clients in identifying problems and discussing several alternative solutions for handling them.

Results of the 1973 study

For the 6 months after discharge from the hospital, the control group's percent time drinking was six times greater, their time spent unemployed was 12 times greater, time spent away from home was twice as high, and time spent institutionalized was 4 times greater than for members of the CRA group. Particularly impressive was the significantly lower percent time drinking for the CRA group (14%) compared to the control group (79%), demonstrating the effectiveness of CRA for the treatment of alcohol problems. The CRA group members received almost twice the controls' mean monthly income and spent more weekends in a structured social activity outside of the home. In summary, the CRA therapy package developed by Hunt and Azrin demonstrated effectiveness in treating problem drinking as well as improving other life areas for members of a traditionally difficult treatment population.

1976: Refining the approach – improvements made in the next trial

The first test of the CRA provided Azrin and his colleagues with promising results concerning its efficacy. It also provided an opportunity to examine and learn from any difficulties encountered during the course of therapy. Building on this knowledge, Azrin implemented several improvements to the program and tested the effectiveness of the new CRA treatment package in a new trial. For example, one problem noted in the original CRA study was the rather lengthy amount of time needed to adequately provide treatment in all its components. To address this issue, the next CRA trial involved counseling clients and their spouses in small groups, and the median time spent in counseling sessions was lowered from 50 hours in the previous trial to 30 hours in the second one. One criticism raised following the original CRA trial was that the counseling was conducted with the efforts of only a single trained therapist. The next trial increased the number of CRA therapists from one to three to test whether each of these individuals could produce positive results using the techniques. Finally, lessons were learned from the initial trial concerning how to better engage clients in new interpersonal relationships and social activities. Overall treatment compliance by both the drinker and his spouse was improved through the use of contracts for taking disulfiram, attending group sessions and marriage counseling, completing the daily reports required in the early warning procedure, and for meeting with the peer advisor.

As in the 1973 trial, Azrin chose as participants 20 hospitalized male clients diagnosed with alcoholism for the 1976 study. Two groups of ten clients were matched on age and education, and on the basis of a life-adjustment score calculated from measures of job satisfaction and stability, family stability, social life, and drinking history. Those randomly assigned to the control group received the regular treatment package provided by the hospital, including instruction regarding alcoholism and its dangers, individual and group counseling, advice to take disulfiram, and encouragement to join an Alcoholics Anonymous group. The remaining participants received these same services in addition to the original CRA procedures and new components included in the revised CRA package: a disulfiram prescription, disulfiram assurance procedures, problem-solving training, a buddy system, and an early warning system.

New CRA treatment components

Disulfiram prescription

An examination of the 1973 results indicated that, while some participants achieved abstinence initially, most had difficulty remaining sober for longer periods. A personal crisis could easily lead to temporary lapses, leaving individuals at greater risk of a full-blown relapse. Azrin and his colleagues needed something to help clients resist the seemingly impulsive urge to return to drinking. With the demonstrated clinical effectiveness of disulfiram (Fox, 1967; Lundwall & Baekeland, 1971), researchers and clinicians had access to a "wonder drug" to deter alcohol use. Disulfiram, marketed as Antabuse®, interferes with the metabolism of alcohol. When taken regularly, the ingestion of alcohol will lead to a physiological reaction, leaving the drinker acutely ill. Azrin reasoned that advocating the use of disulfiram among his clients would prevent the periodic lapses experienced during and after treatment. Also, because clients would have to stop taking disulfiram for a full week before drinking in order to avoid sickness, its regular use would probably eliminate the impulsive drinking seen in response to crises.

Disulfiram assurance procedure

To address the compliance difficulties experienced by treatment providers in the past, Azrin added a "disulfiram assurance" component to the CRA program. Instead of simply describing and prescribing disulfiram, Azrin created additional procedures for motivating clients and training them how to use disulfiram. The procedures ensured that the drinker actually took the disulfiram and was reinforced for doing so.

Azrin noted that alcohol-dependent clients appeared to be resistant to disulfiram use for several reasons. For clients ambivalent about changing their drinking behavior, the idea of taking a drug that would result in extremely negative physical consequences if complete sobriety was not maintained was quite frightening (Azrin, 1976). Some viewed it as a coercive weapon used by doctors to force sobriety on patients, taking away their feelings of choice and control. Others viewed disulfiram use as a crutch which implied that they lacked character or will power. Since negative feelings toward disulfiram could have been partially responsible for a lack of disulfiram compliance, Azrin added motivational procedures to help clients view disulfiram in a positive manner. While describing the disulfiram program to clients, counselors made an effort to describe the medication as a chemical time-delay device which gave the client time to think over a decision rather than to act impulsively. This description emphasized the positive aspect of disulfiram and helped clients to realize that choosing to take the medication could help them take better control of their decisions.

Problems with compliance also occurred when use of disulfiram had not become established as a regular habit. To address this potential difficulty, the client was instructed to ask someone, often a spouse attending sessions, to help him remain sober by monitoring his disulfiram intake every day. The monitor was invited to sessions and guided by the counselor in how to make a positive statement to the client while dispensing the disulfiram, helping the client view the monitor as a caring friend rather than a watchdog. The monitor watched to make sure that the drinker dissolved the disulfiram in liquid and praised the client when he drank the solution, often mentioning how pleased he or she was that the client was making a commitment to work on the drinking problem. The presence of a sober, responsible monitor ensured that daily dosages were more likely to be dispensed and used, getting the client into a regular habit of taking the medication every day.

Problem-solving

In order to help clients prepare for at-risk situations, therapists taught them problem-solving skills based on a modified version of D'Zurilla and Goldfried's (1971) problem-solving approach. Counselors guided the clients through the process of defining the problem, generating acceptable alternatives, deciding on a solution, and later evaluating the outcome. The drinker was asked to review situations from the past that had led to the urge to drink. Through behavioral rehearsal, or role-playing, clients practised acting out trigger situations and handling them in a more adaptive fashion than by resorting to alcohol.

Buddy system

Even though several procedures in the original CRA trial were designed specifically to aid clients in planning for daily nonalcoholic living, many clients still reported difficulties dealing with small hassles and daily issues. Similar to the approach taken in 12-step memberships, a component was added to arrange for a sober "buddy" in the client's neighborhood who could provide advice and support between sessions. The implementation of the buddy system seemed particularly important for clients lacking a social support network. In such cases, this peer advisor also served as the disulfiram monitor and aided the client in other ways, such as providing transportation to the Social Club. The buddy also provided continued social support after counseling had terminated, helping to ensure that improvements would be maintained.

Early warning/mood monitoring

Although disulfiram usage would be a great aid in preventing impulsive slips, Azrin reasoned that clients would also need some assistance in knowing when these slips were likely in order to implement the problem-solving skills that they were learning in the sessions. For this reason, procedures were added to the CRA program to teach the client how to identify and handle danger signals. Specifically, clients and their spouses were instructed to fill out and mail a Happiness Scale to the counselor or peer advisor every day. Spouses had to review and initial each other's Scales on a daily basis prior to mailing them to ensure that potential problems would be communicated to the partner as well as to the counselor. In this way, a homework assignment and support from a spouse aided the clients in recognizing stressors and warning signs even between sessions.

Results of the 1976 study

Follow-up assessments were conducted by a researcher blind to group assignment and extended to a period of 2 years following discharge from the hospital. As in the initial study, the CRA group reported treatment benefits that greatly exceeded those reported by the control group participants (see Table 2.1). At the 6-month follow-up, CRA group members were significantly improved compared to controls in terms of percent time drinking (2% versus 55%), time unemployed (20% versus 56%), time spent away from family (7% versus 67%), and time institutionalized (0% versus 45%). The initial benefits achieved by the CRA group were well maintained for 2 years following the end of treatment, as group members were abstinent for at least 90% of the time for each 6-month follow-up period. It was noteworthy that percent time drinking had lowered from 14% in the Hunt and Azrin (1973) study to 2% in the second study, despite the significant reduction in therapy hours. Finally, each of the three CRA counselors demonstrated the ability to learn and effectively implement the treatment procedures for similar results.

1982: Testing the importance of disulfiram as a CRA component

As Azrin noted when conducting the 1976 study, disulfiram compliance difficulties were a significant barrier in alcohol treatment programs. The major contribution of the study that followed (Azrin et al., 1982) was a test of the relative importance of the disulfiram compliance procedures and the behavioral CRA components introduced in the previous trial. This third examination of CRA was also the first one to test the procedures on an outpatient population and to include female participants. Although it was possible that these outpatient clients would be less severely affected by alcohol problems, it was also a concern that implementing the procedures outside of the structured, contained hospital environment would lead to a lack of participation and treatment compliance. The clients would be expected to face the challenge of confronting their alcohol problems while continuing to live in an old environment that was probably conducive to alcohol abuse. Finally, the 1982 trial allowed Azrin and his colleagues to test the effectiveness of a much abbreviated version of CRA by limiting therapy time to about five hours.

Forty-three outpatient clients diagnosed as alcoholic served as participants in the study. The inclusion criteria stipulated that participants had to be willing and medically able to take disulfiram, had no other drug dependency problems, and were able to have a significant other (i.e., spouse, relative, or close friend) accompany them to the counseling sessions. The mean age of the participants was 33.9 years, 83% were male, 57% were married or cohabiting, and 46% were employed. Average ethanol consumption per drinking day prior to treatment was 264 ml (8.8 ounces), and participants reported an average of 21.1 drinking days per month.

Participants were randomly assigned to one of three treatment groups. Those in the "traditional" (control) group received educational information describing Jellinek's (1960) view of alcoholism and were counseled concerning personal and social problems. Although total abstinence was stressed for members of the traditional group and disulfiram use was encouraged, they did not receive any special disulfiram assurance procedures, and their significant others joined the clients only for the initial session.

The remaining participants were assigned to one of two groups that included a prescription for disulfiram. Those in the "disulfiram assurance" (DA) group received the same treatment plan as the traditional group clients, with the addition of specific training in adhering to the disulfiram regimen. A chosen significant other, often a spouse, was encouraged to accompany the client to all counseling sessions and assisted the client in the daily administration of disulfiram. As in the previous study, regular use of disulfiram was encouraged through role-playing techniques and communication training for clients and spouses.

The third treatment group received the same traditional treatment components and disulfiram assurance procedures mentioned above, yet these clients additionally received a behavioral therapy program. This "behavior therapy plus disulfiram assurance" (CRA + DA) group learned behavioral techniques developed in the CRA trials and were trained in deep muscle relaxation procedures. An important difference between this treatment strategy and the previously described CRA programs was that disulfiram use was not only encouraged but treated as an integral part of the therapy program. Based on results from other studies conducted by Azrin and his colleagues since the 1973 trial, improvements were made in the marital counseling (Azrin, Naster & Jones, 1973; Azrin et al., 1980; Besalel & Azrin, 1981), job finding (Azrin, Flores & Kaplan, 1975; Azrin et al., 1981), and Social Club (Mallams et al., 1982) components. The new treatment techniques tested in the third trial included motivational counseling, sobriety sampling, immediate disulfiram administration, training in drink-refusal skills, and muscle relaxation training. Demonstrating the flexibility inherent in the CRA treatment package, counselors utilized those old and new treatment components which were appropriate for each individual client's needs.

New CRA treatment components

Motivational counseling

To ensure that clients remained motivated to continue with treatment and make important life changes, motivational procedures were developed and implemented. In the first session, clients filled out an *Inconvenience Review Checklist* to indicate the extent of any alcohol-related problems encountered and the clients' current reasons for seeking treatment. Some clients were motivated to quit drinking to receive something pleasant (e.g., feel healthy, obtain a good job), while others were interested in achieving sobriety in order to avoid a negative consequence (e.g., divorce, legal problems). By obtaining this information, counselors were able to refer to these motivators during the course of treatment. If a spouse was present at the first session, the counselor attempted to improve the client's motivation by asking the spouse about negative drinking consequences and his or her personal reasons for wanting the partner to stop drinking. The spouse's observations served as a "reality check" for clients who denied alcohol-related problems, while the spouse's emotional communication of wishes for their relationship served as a powerful reinforcer for change throughout the therapy process. Finally, counselors set positive expectations in their interactions with the clients. They referred to the clients as having "alcohol-related problems" instead of labeling them as "alcoholics", thereby allowing clients to view themselves as individuals capable of changing their behaviors.

Sobriety sampling

For many clients, the thought of never drinking again could be overwhelming (Azrin, 1976). Indeed, a fear that treatment programs would insist on immediate sobriety or hold rigid expectations for the client kept many individuals with drinking problems from entering treatment in the first place. Azrin noted in the 1976 trial that clients often expressed these fears when counselors introduced the notion of taking disulfiram. Although the study's researchers had demonstrated that disulfiram assurance procedures could increase compliance, some clients still voiced their resistance or refused to take the drug altogether. The technique of sobriety sampling was introduced as a relatively nonthreatening option for ambivalent and reluctant individuals. When a client refused to stop drinking or decided against taking disulfiram, the counselor proposed one of several compromises. Clients were asked to consider the possibility of staying abstinent for an agreed-upon, limited period of time in order to simply "sample" sobriety to make a more informed decision about drinking in the future. If possible, clients were also encouraged to sample taking disulfiram during this time. For clients who insisted they could achieve sobriety with will-power alone, the counselor suggested they try their own plan at first but agree to use disulfiram in the future if will-power was not effective enough on its own. Although the ultimate goal for many individuals was life-long abstinence from alcohol, sobriety sampling allowed clients to approach this goal gently, in a less threatening manner.

Sobriety sampling provided many advantages as part of the CRA program. First, the process of working toward a goal together strengthened the counselor–client relationship and allowed the client to feel a sense of choice and control over the treatment process. When clients decided upon goals that were acceptable and likely attainable, they could often have early success experiences that increased their self-confidence and motivation for remaining sober. Upon learning about the client's commitment to a period of sobriety, loved ones became more motivated themselves to provide support and positive reinforcement to the client. Perhaps most importantly, the period of sobriety allowed clients to change old habits and experience the many positive consequences of a nondrinking lifestyle. It was also a test period during which both the client and the therapist could recognize possible barriers to long-term sobriety and implement new coping strategies.

Immediate disulfiram administration

Despite the demonstrated success of the existing disulfiram assurance procedures for encouraging treatment compliance, Azrin et al. (1982) developed yet another way to ensure clients would take the medication. The researchers had noted that motivation for taking disulfiram could easily dissipate soon after the client left the first therapy session. When this occurred, the likelihood that the client would take the initiative to pick up the disulfiram prescription dropped dramatically. Thus, those clients assigned to the disulfiram assurance groups in the 1982 study were guided to obtain the medication immediately after, or even during, the first session. The on-site medical staff were available to hand the client a prescription slip during the first meeting. With a pharmacy within walking distance, clients could fill the prescription immediately and return to the first session ready to take the first dose. Improving access to the medication and assisting the client to take action at a moment of high motivation increased disulfiram compliance even above that witnessed in Azrin and his colleagues' previous work.

Drink refusal

Almost inevitably, drinkers attempting to curb their alcohol use faced pressures from others to return to their former drinking lifestyle. The pressure could be unintentional, such as receiving an invitation from a coworker to attend a party where alcohol would be available. The pressure also could be more blatant, such as a former drinking buddy saying, "So, you think you're too good to drink with me now?" To prepare the client for such situations, Azrin and his colleagues developed drink-refusal training procedures. First, clients were asked to recall situations when they had not wanted to drink but had given in after feeling it was expected of them. Clients' thoughts and feelings about the situation were reviewed, and the counselor suggested they could feel better by deciding to take control of the situation in a more assertive fashion. Clients were instructed to notify friends and family members of their intention to stop drinking and to request that these individuals support them by not offering alcoholic drinks. To prepare for potential awkward or high-risk encounters, counselors helped clients to develop confident responses concerning their decision not to drink and practised them through role-playing.

Muscle relaxation training

An abbreviated form of muscle relaxation training (Azrin, Nunn & Frantz, 1980) was included as a treatment procedure to assist clients in controlling urges to drink. Breathing awareness training, deep muscle relaxation, and instruction in tensing and relaxing individual muscle groups helped clients to achieve physical and mental relaxation. Due to the time limitations imposed by the new five-session format, relaxation training was provided only as needed for those individuals likely to benefit from a reduction in physical tension. These clients often were identified by responses on their *Inconvenience Review Checklist* indicating feelings of anxiety, difficulties sleeping, and physical shakiness.

Results of the 1982 study

To track progress throughout treatment, all clients were taught to record changes in drinking, job performance, arrests, family status, and institutionalization on a monthly calendar that was brought to each treatment session. Additional information was obtained through collateral reports provided by significant others and from in-home follow-up interviews with the clients. At the 6-month follow-up, the three participant groups did not differ significantly on number of days unemployed, days institutionalized, or days away from home. They did, however, differ on number of days taking disulfiram, number of days drinking, amount of alcohol consumed, and number of days intoxicated, with the traditional group faring the worst, the CRA + DA program producing the best results, and the DA group faring somewhere in the middle. During the first month of treatment, clients in all groups were relatively sober, but the differences between the groups became greater with each passing month. In the final month of the 6-month follow-up, the abstinence rates for the traditional, the DA, and the CRA + DA groups were 45%, 74%, and 97%, respectively.

Two results in particular were noteworthy. While CRA group participants in the 1976 study received a median of 30 treatment hours to reduce their drinking time to 2%, participants receiving disulfiram and a similar behavioral CRA treatment in the 1982 study had reduced their drinking to a similar level at the 6-month follow-up after attending an average of only 6.4 sessions. Another interesting result of the 1982 study was the finding of an interaction between the effectiveness of a particular treatment package and the marital status of the client. For married clients, the disulfiram assurance procedures provided as many benefits as did the full CRA program, but single clients gained more if they received the full CRA program than if they simply received the DA intervention. Therefore, a less intensive, and perhaps less expensive, set of procedures could be effectively utilized for achieving sobriety for drinkers in relationships with romantic partners who could assist in assuring disulfiram compliance. The 1982 study was one of the few existing verifications at the time of the effectiveness of disulfiram in alcohol treatment. By including behavioral procedures to assure that the drinker actually took the drug daily, the effectiveness of its use could be evaluated without the usual problem of client drop-out or noncompliance.

The legacy of Azrin's early CRA studies

Over the years, CRA has proven to be an intense treatment that is able to improve many areas in a person's life in as little as 4–6 weeks and with as few as five sessions. The creation of a treatment "package" proved to be important for individuals with familial, social, and employment problems as well as chronic alcohol problems. In addition, the ability to use or not use particular components has allowed counselors to tailor treatment to an individual's needs. The resulting therapy approach could be utilized for the goal of achieving life-long abstinence from alcohol as well as for helping clients interested in moderation.

At the time of its development, CRA was unique in its emphasis on recognizing the important impact of an individual's environment, both for encouraging and for discouraging drinking behavior. In particular, Azrin and his colleagues realized the treatment benefits possible by actively involving an invested significant other in the drinker's treatment plan. The flexible CRA procedures were also able to accommodate the needs of individuals who lacked an environment with supportive loved ones and nondrinking activities by creating synthetic families and providing a peer advisor and a Social Club to build new friendships. Support for a client's sobriety continued between therapy sessions when clients were encouraged to use techniques learned from the counselor and to take advantage of the availability of provided resources (e.g., the peer advisor and Social Club) in his or her environment. It quickly became clear that CRA was unique among treatment approaches in that the counselors involved themselves personally and directly in the client's treatment, at times going beyond the boundaries of the therapy session to accompany the client to job interviews or help in other capacities.

Since the publication of the 1982 study, Azrin and other researchers have continued to refine and test the CRA treatment program for substance abuse treatment. These researchers also sought to address some important limitations and criticisms of Azrin's earlier work (*see* Chapter 4). The effectiveness of the CRA procedures has now been demonstrated with a broader range of participant groups, including adolescent drug abusers (Azrin et al., 1994, 1996), cocaine abusers (Budney et al., 1991; Higgins et al., 1991, 1993*a*, *b*), and homeless men and women dependent on alcohol (Smith, Meyers & Delaney, 1998). The observation of the effectiveness of spousal involvement in therapy and the fact that many substance abusers were resistant to treatment led to the creation of a "reinforcement training" program for spouses and family members of treatment-resistant substance users (Meyers, Dominguez & Smith, 1996; Sisson & Azrin, 1986). Its potential flexibility and common-sense techniques suggest that CRA may be extended to clients in a broad range of age groups and with varying presenting problems. Such investigations are continuing nearly three decades since Hunt and Azrin introduced the scientific treatment community to the CRA.

3

The Treatment

JANE ELLEN SMITH AND ROBERT J. MEYERS

Overview

This chapter outlines the components of the CRA treatment program (see Meyers & Smith, 1995, for complete details). The assessment and treatment planning techniques are utilized with all clients, but a client's particular behavioral deficits dictate which skills training procedures are introduced.

Community Reinforcement Approach functional analyses

Although behavior therapists may already use functional analyses as a standard part of their treatment for various types of disturbed behavior, they are still a relatively rare tool as far as substance-abuse programs are concerned. A traditional functional analysis is a semi-structured interview which outlines the antecedents (triggers) and consequences of a specific behavior. Its purpose is to diagram the context in which the behavior is occurring. Once the *triggers* for the behavior are identified, we typically assist in the development of a plan either to avoid these high-risk situations, or to acquire the necessary skills for addressing them. As far as examining the *consequences* of a problem behavior is concerned, this information is critical for determining the role that the behavior is serving. The Community Reinforcement Approach (CRA) functional analysis first looks at the positive consequences, since these are the factors that maintain the behavior. Eventually we work with the client to realize healthier ways to obtain these positive consequences. The negative consequences of the problem behavior are outlined so that the client clearly sees the price that is being paid for the behavior. It also provides us with a list of the people and opportunities that are important to the client and which have been lost or jeopardized because of the problem behavior. This information can later be used to motivate the client to make sound decisions.

One of the unique features of the CRA functional analysis is that both drinking (or drug-using) *and* pleasurable, nonproblematic behaviors are examined routinely, with the goal of decreasing the substance-abusing behavior and increasing the nonproblematic behavior. To simplify the language in this chapter, problem drinking is used as an example of substance-abusing behavior. With this in mind, the drinking behavior is outlined first. We begin by asking the client to describe a common drinking scenario. If the client reports that there are several common ones, we ask the client either to select the one that occurs most often, or the one most likely to present itself in the upcoming week. We listen carefully to the description of the event, while jotting down pertinent facts on a CRA Functional Analysis For Drinking Behavior Chart (see Figure 3.1). Once the client finishes the description, we return to the "trigger" columns on the chart and pose questions until the antecedents for the drinking episode are clearly outlined.

The first column covers "external" triggers, or environmental factors, such as people, places, and times associated with alcohol use in that episode. And so, if it has not already been covered, we ask, "*Who* are you usually with when you drink? *Where* and *when* do you drink?" Assume, for example, that a male client is discussing a typical weekend scenario in which he works hard on the house and yard all day Saturday, and then heads over to a friend's to play cards and drink in the evening. Also assume that he has a beer or two while doing the yard work, but, according to his report, the drinking does not get out of hand until he is playing cards. We would make a note of the drinking that occurs earlier in the day, as it may actually set the stage for the later excessive drinking, and consequently might need to be addressed. But for now the evening episode alone will be the focus, since the client has identified this as a problem on which he would like to work. In terms of the CRA Functional Analysis For Drinking Behavior Chart, the external triggers for the episode are known already (see Figure 3.2 for an example of a chart completed for this client).

Once the high-risk environmental context is outlined, we move on to explore internal triggers. These are the thoughts, physical sensations, and emotions that set the stage for the drinking episode. Imagine, for example, that this client reports feeling physically exhausted but very pleased with himself on these Saturdays when he has worked so hard. His thoughts are along the line of, "I need to relax" and "I deserve a little bit of fun after

CRA Functional Analysis for Drinking Behavior (Initial Assessment)

External triggers	Internal triggers	Drinking behavior	Short-term positive consequences	Long-term negative consequences
1. *Who* are you usually with when you drink?	1. What are you usually *thinking* about right before you drink?	1. *What* do you usually drink?	1. What do you like about drinking with (*who*)?	1. What are the negative results of your drinking in each of these areas:
2. *Where* do you usually drink?	2. What are you usually *feeling physically* right before you drink?	2. *How much* do you usually drink?	2. What do you like about drinking (*where*)?	a. Interpersonal b. Physical c. Emotional d. Legal
3. *When* do you usually drink?	3. What are you usually *feeling emotionally* right before you drink?	3. Over *how long* a period of time do you usually drink?	3. What do you like about drinking (*when*)?	

4. What are the pleasant
   thoughts you have
   while drinking?

   e. Job
   f. Financial
   g. Other

5. What are the pleasant
   physical feelings you
   have while drinking?

6. What are the pleasant
   emotions you have
   while drinking?

Figure 3.1 CRA Functional Analysis for Drinking Behavior (Initial Assessment). From *Clinical guide to alcohol treatment: the Community Reinforcement Approach* by R. J. Meyers & J. E. Smith, 1995, pp. 34–35. Copyright 1995 by Guilford Press, New York. Adapted with permission.

CRA Functional Analysis for Drinking Behavior (Initial Assessment)

External triggers	Internal triggers	Drinking behavior	Short-term positive consequences	Long-term negative consequences
1. *Who* are you usually with when you drink? *Marcello, Dale and James.*	1. What are you usually *thinking* about right before you drink? *I need to relax.* *I deserve some fun for working so hard.* *I'll fit in because I'll be drinking.*	1. *What* do you usually drink? *Beer.*	1. What do you like about drinking with (*who*)? *We laugh a lot.* *They think I'm funny.*	1. What are the negative results of your drinking in each of these areas: a. Interpersonal *I only seem to have friends who drink. I haven't put any effort into find up a romantic relationship lately.*
2. *Where* do you usually drink? *Marcello's house.*	2. What are you usually *feeling physically* right before you drink? *Exhausted.*	2. *How much* do you usually drink? *7–8 12-oz. bottles.*	2. What do you like about drinking (*where*)? *I don't have to drive far.* *It's informal; I can be myself.*	b. Physical *I don't sleep well Saturday night, and I feel low energy Sunday.* c. Emotional *I feel lonely; I don't know if it's related to drinking.*
3. *When* do you usually drink? *Saturday night.*	3. What are you usually *feeling emotionally* right before you drink? *Pleased with self.* *A little sad.*	3. Over *how long* a period of time do you usually drink? *3 hours.*	3. What do you like about drinking (*when*)? *It's a good way to unwind after working all day.*	d. Legal *No problems, but I worry about getting a DWI.*

4. What are the pleasant *thoughts* you have while drinking?
These guys think I'm funny and they like me around.

5. What are the pleasant *physical feelings* you have while drinking?
I feel relaxed.

6. What are the pleasant *emotions* you have while drinking?
Feeling "high", happy, content.

e. Job
The Saturday drinking doesn't affect this, but my weekday drinking may be starting to.

f. Financial
No problem here.

g. Other
n/a

Figure 3.2 CRA Functional Analysis for Drinking Behavior (Initial Assessment). Sample of completed form.

working so hard today." We enter these on the chart and probe for additional internal triggers. Assume the client also states that he sometimes feels a little sad because he thinks he only really fits in with these friends when he is drinking. We accept the client's thoughts and feelings that are associated with the excessive drinking, and briefly explain how therapy will focus on finding healthier options for relaxing and having fun after a hard day's work. We also make a note about eventually needing to focus on this client's nondrinking social activities and friendships.

The middle segment of the CRA functional analysis entails gathering basic quantity and frequency information about the drinking behavior. The severity of the alcohol problem can often be gleaned from this, and progress can be monitored by referring back to these data throughout treatment. If the client has already given this information in the course of generally describing the episode, we simply review it briefly right after discussing the triggers, so that the link between the triggers and the drinking is emphasized. As noted on the chart (see Figure 3.2), the client reported drinking about seven to eight bottles of beer during a three-hour period.

The last part of the CRA functional analysis examines the consequences of the drinking behavior. It is important to acknowledge the positive effects, since these are the factors that are maintaining the behavior. At the same time, their short-lived nature should be pointed out. The ultimate goal is to acknowledge the function of the drinking, and eventually to work toward finding alternate routes to those same outcomes, or to modify a series of behaviors so that the outcomes are no longer needed. In the case of our client who drinks on Saturday nights, assume that his short-term positive consequences are those listed in the fourth column of Figure 3.2. In other words, the drinking is associated with a comfortable social atmosphere in which he can relax and be happy. We note that social acceptance seems important to him ("These guys think I'm funny and they like me around"), and we plan again to later explore nondrinking options for relaxing and socializing.

The final piece of the CRA functional analysis used for the drinking behavior is an exploration of the negative consequences. In all probability the client has mentioned a number of these already, but it is useful to inquire about each of the areas listed: interpersonal, physical, emotional, legal, job, and financial. Our current client appeared most concerned about his lack of close interpersonal relationships, and the role that his drinking might be playing. He also commented on his weekday drinking, which certainly would be explored in a second functional analysis at a later time.

CRA offers a unique second type of functional analysis: one for pleasurable nondrinking behaviors (see Figure 3.3). One purpose of this exercise is to highlight the fact that the client is already engaging in enjoyable activities that do not involve alcohol. Eventually we encourage the client to increase the frequency of participation in these or other pleasurable, alcohol-free activities. But in order to set the stage to do this, the functional analysis is needed to outline both the common precursors for this behavior as well as some of the unfavorable consequences. Since in this situation the goal is to increase the chance that this behavior will occur, we teach the client to recognize these triggers and to respond more regularly to them with a healthy behavior. Also, in a subsequent session we teach problem-solving skills in an effort to reduce any of the minimally negative consequences associated with the mostly pleasurable activities.

Most drinkers have had innumerable people, including therapists, dwell on all of the enjoyable, alcohol-related behaviors that they should *stop* doing. So it comes as a welcome surprise to have a therapist explain how it is equally important to spend time discussing ways to introduce pleasant activities that can compete with and replace drinking behaviors. With this in mind, we invite the client to select one pleasurable, nondrinking activity that is already in his or her behavioral repertoire. We then have the client describe the external and internal triggers that set the stage for this behavior. Assume that the client introduced earlier says he wants to go on a dinner and movie date for his pleasurable activity. Since upon questioning it becomes clear that the client does not currently even have a particular female in mind, we decide to have him first select an activity that is more readily available and under his control. The client next suggests that he could do the same activity with his sister, but since they argue a lot it might not be consistently enjoyable. We encourage the client to search for yet another option, because the activity certainly would have to be pleasant in order to compete with his card playing and drinking. The client settles on going to his brother's house for dinner and a video, where he can enjoy time with his two young nephews. Upon learning that the brother and sister-in-law do not drink, we support this choice for an activity, since it does not place the client in a high-risk situation, it seems feasible, and it is available during a high-risk time.

CRA Functional Analysis for Nondrinking Behavior

External triggers	Internal triggers	Nondrinking behavior	Short-term negative consequences	Long-term positive consequences
1. *Who* are you usually with when you (*activity*)?	1. What are you usually *thinking* about right before you (*activity*)?	1. *What* is the nondrinking activity?	1. What do you dislike about (*activity*) with (*who*)?	1. What are the positive results of your (*activity*) in each of these areas: a. Interpersonal b. Physical c. Emotional d. Legal
2. *Where* do you usually (*activity*)?	2. What are you usually *feeling physically* right before you (*activity*)?	2. *How often* do you engage in it?	2. What do you dislike about (*activity*) (*where*)?	
3. *When* do you usually (*activity*)?	3. What are you usually *feeling emotionally* right before you (*activity*)?	3. How *long* does it usually last?	3. What do you dislike about (*activity*) (*when*)?	

4. What are the
unpleasant *thoughts*
you have while
(*activity*)?

5. What are the
unpleasant *physical
feelings* you have while
(*activity*)?

6. What are the
unpleasant *emotions*
you have while
(*activity*)?

e. Job
f. Financial
g. Other

Figure 3.3 CRA Functional Analysis for Nondrinking Behavior. From *Clinical guide to alcohol treatment: the Community Reinforcement Approach* by R. J. Meyers & J. E. Smith, 1995, pp. 38–39. Copyright 1995 by Guilford Press, New York. Adapted with permission.

CRA Functional Analysis for Nondrinking Behavior

External triggers	Internal triggers	Nondrinking behavior	Short-term negative consequences	Long-term positive consequences
1. *Who* are you usually with when you (*activity*)? *My brother Charles, his wife Jill, and their 2 boys.*	1. What are you usually *thinking* about right before you (*activity*)? *This is a good way to spend the evening. It's something to do. It's nice to get to know my nephews. I hope nobody bugs me about my social life.*	1. *What* is the nondrinking activity? *Dinner at brother's house: video afterwards.*	1. What do you dislike about (*activity*) with (*who*)? *It gets really noisy sometimes. Once in a while I get interrogated about whether I'm dating.*	1. What are the positive results of your (*activity*) in each of these areas: a. Interpersonal *It brings me closer to my family; I get to be a part of my nephews' lives.* b. Physical *It's healthier than drinking all night.* c. Emotional *My nephews look up to me and are always thrilled to see me; that feels really good.* d. Legal *No chance of a DWI.*
2. *Where* do you usually (*activity*)? *Their house.*	2. What are you usually feeling physically right before you (*activity*)? *Tired.*	2. *How often* do you engage in it? *About once a month.*	2. What do you dislike about (*activity*) (*where*)? *Nothing.*	
3. *When* do you usually (*activity*)? *They invite me most Saturday nights. I go only occasionally.*	3. What are you usually feeling emotionally right before you (*activity*)? *Content, but a little disappointed that I won't be drinking ... and then ashamed for feeling that.*	3. How *long* does it usually last? *About 3 hours.*	3. What do you dislike about (*activity*) (*when*)? *It's just not as much fun as drinking and playing cards.*	

4. What are the unpleasant thoughts you have while (activity)?

Am I ever going to have my own family? I'm getting old and time is passing me by.

5. What are the unpleasant physical feelings you have while (activity)?

My stomach gets upset sometimes because I eat so much there.

6. What are the unpleasant emotions you have while (activity)?

Disappointment in myself for not having things together in my life

e. Job

My brother and his wife help me sort out job-related problems.

f. Financial

I don't lose money like I do at cards.

g. Other

Figure 3.4 CRA Functional Analysis for Nondrinking Behavior. Sample of completed form.

In exploring the triggers for eating dinner at his brother's house, we listen for signs that can be turned into cues to select this activity over cards and drinking. For example, assume the client states that typically before going to his brother's house he thinks about how it is at least something to do socially, and that he enjoys getting to know his nephews better (see Figure 3.4). When it later becomes time to discuss plans for increasing this activity, we will ask him to focus on thoughts about his nephews and why he likes to be around them, since attention to the social aspects could easily steer him toward the card game instead. For now, we listen for any ambivalent feelings that may precede the dinner decision, and which consequently could act as a deterrent. In this case the client reports that sometimes he feels hassled about his social life by his brother when he visits, and this is unpleasant since he is not dating. We might introduce social skills training or problem-solving to address this issue if it appears warranted.

Often the column for describing the nondrinking behavior has already been completed at this point in the functional analysis, and so we move to the short-term negative consequences. Not surprisingly, many pleasurable activities have some aversive components that, at times, interfere with the decision to select that activity. The functional analysis helps sort out these factors by specifically inquiring about the client's negative thoughts and feelings both during and immediately following the behavior of interest. In the current case, the client's main sources of discomfort are disappointment in himself for not having his life "together", and the fear that he never will have his own family. We reassure the client that problems in other areas of his life will be the focus of treatment as well. Deterrents requiring immediate attention are addressed through problem-solving (see "Behavioral skills training" section).

As far as identifying the long-term positive consequences for the non-drinking behavior, the same categories are presented as for the drinking chart. In this situation we take note of the client's reinforcers, so that they can be incorporated in subsequent sessions and presented as reasons to pursue a healthier lifestyle. So assume the client reports that both interpersonal and emotional benefits are associated with having dinner at his brother's house. We do not shy away from suggesting other possible reinforcing aspects of the behavior, since activities that are seen as rewarding in many different areas of the client's life will probably be good candidates for behaviors that compete with drinking. Eventually we will ask the client to plan additional recreational activities with other individuals, particularly nondrinkers, who can offer benefits similar to those outlined in the long-term positive consequences column of his chart. Furthermore, therapy time will be devoted to addressing the obstacles preventing him from having his own romantic relationship.

Although functional analyses for drinking and nondrinking behaviors are always completed at the beginning of CRA treatment, they are referred to throughout the program and new ones are introduced as needed. Sometimes we send copies of the charts home with clients to serve as reminders of high-risk situations and their warning signals, or, in the case of the nondrinking charts, to prompt them to select behaviors that compete with drinking.

Sobriety sampling

Many traditional alcohol treatment programs in the United States use abstinence as their only drinking goal. Consequently, clients are told from the start that they can *never* drink again. As noted previously, this is experienced as an extremely threatening message by many individuals, particularly those who are not convinced that they even have a drinking problem. Not surprisingly, a high percentage of them respond by never returning to treatment. The CRA program's sobriety sampling procedure approaches the goals of treatment in a much gentler way. It operates on the assumption that clients will be more successfully engaged in therapy if they are not overwhelmed by rigid rules and frightening expectations. And so sobriety sampling is a negotiation process between the therapist and the client in which a commitment to a limited period of abstinence is agreed upon. Regardless of whether the ultimate goal is abstinence or moderate drinking, at least a limited period of abstinence at the start of treatment is encouraged for all.

In introducing the notion of sampling sobriety, some of the specific advantages of a "time-out" from drinking are presented:

1. It allows the client to experience the sensation of being sober on a daily basis. After a rough initial period, this usually focuses attention automatically on positive changes in cognitive, emotional, and physical symptoms.
2. It is viewed by family members as a commitment to change, which in turn elicits their support.
3. It prevents the reliance on drinking as a coping strategy, and instead gives the client the opportunity to substitute new coping behaviors.

4. It affords the client some practice in setting and achieving manageable goals, which then works to enhance self-esteem and confidence.
5. In the event that the client experiences difficulty in maintaining sobriety during this monitored period, it provides valuable information regarding troublesome areas.

Once a client agrees to sample sobriety, a reasonable period of time must be selected. We begin by suggesting a relatively lengthy period, such as 90 days, with the understanding that this will leave plenty of room for negotiation downward. The suggestion is backed by the rationale that the first 90 days appears to be the time during which most relapses occur (Marlatt & Gordon, 1985). Perhaps not surprisingly, most clients report that they are unwilling or unable to make a 90-day commitment. We do not interpret this as resistance, but instead work with the client to select a shorter time period that appears challenging yet obtainable. Whenever possible, the client's reinforcers are introduced to provide an added incentive. For example, assume a female drinker has reported during her functional analysis that one of the negative interpersonal consequences associated with her alcohol use is that her son does not like her to spend time with his children when she is drinking. As a result, invitations to the son's house have grown infrequent. We would inquire about any upcoming special functions with the grandchildren, and would attempt to link them to a period of sobriety. For instance, if the client's granddaughter's birthday was in 5 weeks, we would actively encourage the client to settle upon a time commitment that took her through that date.

Regardless of the length of the negotiated period of sobriety, we assist the client in devising a plan for accomplishing this at least until the necessary skills can be taught. Typically we refer to the client's triggers on the functional analysis, and then help to identify behaviors that compete with drinking in those high-risk situations. Problem-solving training is often introduced at this point as well. Finally, sessions are scheduled several times per week during this stage in therapy, so that the client has the opportunity to quickly learn the skills needed to honor the sobriety commitment. Assuming a client reaches the negotiated sobriety goal, we discuss the advantages of sampling sobriety for an additional limited period. Ideally those reinforcers that are already being received by the client for being abstinent serve as an incentive.

Monitored disulfiram

Some clients experience great difficulty achieving a period of abstinence early in treatment, despite their professed desire to do so. For these individuals, the addition of disulfiram to their treatment program may be a reasonable option. Disulfiram (Antabuse®) is a medication that acts as a deterrent to drinking, since the ingestion of any alcohol while taking disulfiram causes an aversive chemical reaction. Depending on a number of factors, this may range from feeling mildly sick to requiring emergency medical attention. So although disulfiram can be an extremely effective adjunct to treatment, it obviously only works if individuals agree to take it in the first place, and then only as long as they remain on it.

Individuals who appear to be good candidates for disulfiram are presented with its pros and cons. The advantages include:

1. A decrease in complicated, agonizing daily decisions about drinking, because there is only one decision to make each day: whether or not to take the pill.
2. A reduction in "slips" that result from impulsive drinking, since it remains in one's system for up to 2 weeks after it is discontinued.
3. An increase in the ability to address many drinking triggers at once, since the triggers lose their power if drinking simply is not an option.
4. An increase in family trust and a decrease in family worry, as significant others feel confident that their loved one is not drinking.
5. An increase in opportunities for positive reinforcement, since at the very least the client is praised daily by the monitor who is administering the disulfiram.

If the client agrees to take disulfiram it must first be medically cleared. The next step is to identify a monitor, who is a readily available concerned family member or friend. The job of the monitor is to administer the disulfiram to the client daily in a supportive manner. Having a monitor is an essential component of the disulfiram procedure (Azrin et al., 1982). The monitor is invited to a therapy session so that he or she can be trained to communicate with the client during the daily disulfiram administration in a manner that is positively reinforcing. For example, the monitor is taught to hand the disulfiram to the drinker and say, "I really appreciate you taking your disulfiram again. I know it must be hard to do. It shows me how committed you are to stopping drinking." The client receives training in how to reply in a supportive manner as well. And since this type of conversation is not typically a natural one, it is role-played several times during the session and feedback is provided. The client and monitor are then asked to select a time and place to take the disulfiram daily, so as to establish a routine (see Meyers & Smith, 1995, pp. 72–73 for a complete description).

Most clients do not remain on disulfiram for more than a few months. This tends to be sufficient time to teach problem drinkers the necessary skills to support a nondrinking lifestyle. Also, the reinforcement received from family and friends during this alcohol-free period supports continued sobriety.

CRA treatment plan

The foundation of CRA's behavioral treatment plan is built on two instruments: The Happiness Scale and the Goals of Counseling form. The Happiness Scale is a one-page questionnaire that asks about an individual's current level of happiness in ten categories: drinking, job/educational progress, money management, social life, personal habits, marriage/family relationships, legal issues, emotional life, communication, and general happiness (see Figure 3.5). The client circles a number from 1 (completely unhappy) to 10 (completely happy) for each category. The Happiness Scale provides a precounseling baseline of dissatisfaction across a variety of problem areas, and subsequent administrations of it allow us to monitor progress. In completing this form clients recognize that therapy will focus on other important areas of their lives in addition to the substance use.

Once problem areas are identified, the next step involves setting behavioral goals and devising the plans for achieving them. The Goals of Counseling form provides a useful framework for this exercise, as it includes the same ten categories listed on the Happiness Scale. As with most behavioral plans, brief and measurable terms are used when specifying both the goals and the intervention strategies. Whenever possible, emphasis is also placed on stating goals in a positive manner; namely, what the client *will* do, as opposed to what he or she will *not* do anymore. In most cases clients appear to know what they should *stop* doing, but they often are unaware of how best to replace the behavior. And since they have difficulty formulating measurable behaviors as well, we spend time shaping the goals. For example, assume a client wishes to work on improving his social life. A common first attempt at stating this goal is, "I want to stop hanging out at bars all the time." We reinforce the client's efforts in

Happiness Scale

This scale is intended to estimate your *current* happiness with your life in each of the ten areas listed below. Ask yourself the following question as you rate each area:

How happy am I with this area of my life?

You are to circle one of the numbers (1–10) beside each area.

Numbers toward the left indicate various degrees of unhappiness, while numbers toward the right reflect various levels of happiness.

In other words, state according to the numerical scale (1–10) exactly how you feel today.

Remember: Try to exclude all feelings of yesterday and concentrate only on the feelings of today in each of the life areas. Also try not to allow one category to influence the results of the other categories.

	Completely unhappy						Completely happy			
Drinking	1	2	3	4	5	6	7	8	9	10
Job or education progress	1	2	3	4	5	6	7	8	9	10
Money management	1	2	3	4	5	6	7	8	9	10
Social life	1	2	3	4	5	6	7	8	9	10
Personal habits	1	2	3	4	5	6	7	8	9	10
Marriage/family relationships	1	2	3	4	5	6	7	8	9	10
Legal issues	1	2	3	4	5	6	7	8	9	10
Emotional life	1	2	3	4	5	6	7	8	9	10
Communication	1	2	3	4	5	6	7	8	9	10
General happiness	1	2	3	4	5	6	7	8	9	10

Name:_____   Date:_____

Figure 3.5 Happiness Scale. From *Clinical guide to alcohol treatment: the Community Reinforcement Approach* by R. J. Meyers & J. E. Smith, 1995, p. 95. Copyright 1995 by Guilford Press, New York. Adapted with permission.

general, and the fact that the goal was worded briefly. Guidance is provided to redefine the goal in positive, measurable terms, such as, "I will participate in one new, nondrinking social activity each week for the next month." (See Figure 3.6 for a sample page from a completed Goals of Counseling form for this client.)

Specific strategies for achieving the goals are identified next. Depending on the individual's skills, several steps may need to be outlined. For instance, the client may first require a plan for identifying some potentially enjoyable alcohol-free activities, and then encouragement to involve a friend. We next determine if there appear to be any obstacles to implementing the plan, and, if so, we address them. Progress toward the goal is checked in the next session. Additional reasonable goals in other problem areas can also be established in the initial session if the client's level of functioning permits. Several examples are listed in Figure 3.6.

Use of the CRA treatment plan is similar to the functional analysis inasmuch as it is referred to and modified throughout treatment. Not only do clients' goals change as therapy progresses, but the strategies available to them for achieving the goals diversify as clients acquire behavioral skills.

Behavioral skills training

An essential component of the CRA program involves identifying behavioral skill deficits, and then providing training to improve those skills. The particular deficits are uncovered in a variety of ways. Some are illuminated through conversations with the client, and others surface as obstacles when working toward specific goals on the Goals of Counseling form. Finally, we sometimes find it useful to return to the functional analysis to review the role served by the drinking. If the drinking is maintained by positive reinforcement, we determine whether the client has the behavioral repertoire to obtain positive reinforcement through healthier means. For example, if the drinking is experienced as enjoyable because it provides the opportunity to socialize, we assess whether the client possesses the *communication skills* to meet new, nondrinking friends. In the event that the client is already reasonably socially skillful, but is uncertain how to find nondrinking friends, *problem-solving* training is indicated instead. Alternatively, if the client is willing to seek new social outlets, but his or her unassertive style is a risk factor for drinking if alcohol is offered, then *drink-refusal* training is given. For cases in which the drinking is maintained by negative reinforcement, such as decreasing stress and anxiety, we

Goals of Counseling

Name: _____

Date: _____

Problem areas/goals	Intervention	Time frame
4. In the area of social life I would like:		
To participate in 1 new nondrinking social activity each week.	a. Look through newspaper 2x/week and circle interesting activities that are alcohol free.	1 month.
	b. Call a friend and invite him/her to one of the activities. Make specific plans to attend.	
5. In the area of personal habits I would like:		
a. To clean my apartment at least every other week.	A a. Clean bathroom the 1st and 3rd Saturdays of the month.	Ongoing every 2 weeks.
	b. Clean kitchen, living room, bedroom the 2nd and 4th Saturdays.	
b. To wash my dishes daily.	B. Wash dishes immediately after using them, or rinse and load in dishwasher.	Ongoing daily.
6. In the area of marriage/family relationships I would like:		
To have a meal with my parents once a week.	a. Call my mom Friday or Saturday and ask about joining them for a meal Sunday or Monday.	Ongoing 1x/week.
	b. Ask if there's anything she needs me to do for her before then.	

Figure 3.6 Goals of Counseling. Sample of completed form.

ascertain whether the client needs problem-solving training to assist in generating other feasible options for alleviating stress.

In terms of *communication skills training*, the CRA program focuses on increasing positive interchanges by relying on seven basic guidelines. Although these guidelines can be successfully applied to most conversations, they are particularly helpful for those involving discussions of problems. They are taught because they offer a precise communication in a manner that minimizes a defensive reaction from the listener. The steps are:

1. Be brief.
2. Be positive.
3. Use specific (measurable) terms.
4. Label your feelings.
5. Give an understanding statement.
6. Accept partial responsibility.
7. Offer to help.

In presenting these steps we point out that the first three should look familiar, as they provided the framework for formulating goals and strategies on the treatment plan. Steps 4 and 5 are seen as complementary, since one is a comment about the client's feelings, while the understanding statement introduces empathy. Additionally, clients are encouraged to make a partial responsibility statement as a way of acknowledging a role in creating the problem. The final step, offering to help, is viewed as a positive first step toward problem-solving. Not surprisingly, some clients express resentment when asked to practise the last two steps, particularly if they believe that they are not at all responsible for the problem. We remind these clients that communication can only be effective if the other person listens to it, and that the last two steps play an important role in facilitating this.

Educating a client about the components of a good conversation is only the beginning. Assume a client's first attempt at asking her husband to turn the TV down at night once she is in bed sounds like, "Honey, I'm really tired of begging you to turn the TV down every night. How would *you* like it if I did something that interfered with your sleep?" We reinforce the client for being brief and for labeling her feelings, and we then model an improved conversation that incorporates several more steps from the guidelines. With repeated practice, the final conversation approximates the following, "Honey, I know that you've gotten used to staying up late and watching TV over the years (understanding statement). And I know that when I was drinking I wasn't good company anyway (partial responsibility). But it upsets me now when you leave the volume up loud after 11:00 p.m., because it's hard for me to fall asleep (feelings; specific terms). I wouldn't mind checking into getting you a set of headphones for the TV (offer to help; positive terms). What do you think?"

Many clients improve markedly throughout the training process, but others are only able to incorporate a few of the steps into their conversations. Regardless, all clients are verbally rewarded for their efforts, and are informed that the use of even just one or two new steps is probably an improvement over previous communications. Generalization of skills into the real world is monitored.

The second part of CRA's behavioral skills program is *problem-solving training*. A modified version of D'Zurilla and Goldfried's (1971) approach is utilized. The purpose of the procedure is to teach clients a new appropriate strategy for coping with stressors without resorting to alcohol use. The steps are as follows:

1. Define the problem. The client identifies the problem, and we help modify the description so that it is stated clearly and in very specific terms.
2. Brainstorm possible solutions. The client is instructed to begin generating a list of potential solutions to the problem. We ensure that none of the ideas will be criticized or questioned. All suggestions are written down for the client to see. Usually at least ten suggestions are expected, and so we assist by offering a few ideas if necessary.
3. Eliminate undesired solutions. The client is invited next to cross out any solutions that he or she cannot imagine trying in the upcoming week. Explanations are not required.
4. Select one potential solution. The client is asked to review the remaining solutions, to select one, and to make a commitment to trying it prior to the next session.
5. Generate possible obstacles. We instruct the client to consider potential obstacles in the upcoming week that might interfere with carrying out the selected solution. Common examples may be given: forgetting, becoming too busy.
6. Devise a plan for each obstacle. The client is asked to devise a specific plan for addressing each obstacle. If this proves difficult to do, the client is encouraged to select a different solution.

7. Evaluate the effectiveness of the solution. At the next session we inquire if the solution was attempted, and, if so, how well it worked. Frequently the solution needs to be modified somewhat, and at times a new solution is decided upon instead.

Problem-solving training is an excellent mechanism for addressing stressors in a wide variety of areas. It is critical for clients to have such a tool, because it minimizes the chance that they will again rely on escaping through alcohol use. It is also essential for clients to practise applying it to real-life issues as they occur, so we make every effort to introduce problem-solving during sessions whenever a current problem is raised by the client. For instance, if a client arrives 20 minutes late for a session and explains that he is having trouble getting a ride, we help him use the problem-solving procedure to generate a solution to the transportation problem.

The third major component of CRA's behavioral skills training is *drink refusal*. There are several segments to this program, with the first involving the enlistment of social support from the client's "community". And so the client is asked to inform family members and close friends that he or she is no longer drinking. The belief is that if a client's "community" reinforces nondrinking behavior, then the client is more likely to continue engaging in it. The second part of drink-refusal training entails reviewing high-risk drinking situations. The CRA Functional Analysis For Drinking Behavior Chart can be referred to here, as the triggers for at least one common episode are outlined. However, the client is also asked to generate a list of five to ten typical scenarios in which a slip is possible. Depending on the situation and the client's skill level, he or she may be advised to avoid it altogether, or to assertively refuse alcohol if it is offered.

Teaching a client how to refuse alcohol in an assertive manner is the third component of CRA's drink-refusal training. The work of Monti et al. (1989) is relied upon heavily when illustrating options for turning down alcohol. But again, educating a client is only the first step. Behavior rehearsal through role-plays is essential. The basic options presented are:

1. Saying, "No, thanks."
2. Suggesting alternative beverages.
3. Changing the subject.
4. Questioning the aggressor.

The simplistic sounding "just say no" option is raised because many clients assume that they owe individuals an explanation for refusing alcohol.

Since turning down a drink feels foreign to them, they believe that others will perceive it that way also. After a short discussion of the topic, relatively assertive clients are invited to try it for a week, and to report the consequences in the next session. Many clients require additional choices though, and so option number 2 is presented and practised. For example, a client might be taught to say, "Actually, I'd love a strong cup of coffee instead." The third suggestion, which involves raising a new topic, is a distraction technique. The client might prepare a line such as, "No, thanks. I really don't feel like having a beer tonight. Hey, which teams do you think are going to make it to the finals this season?" Typically the fourth and final option is reserved for situations in which the client is being pressured to drink despite having executed options 1–3 already. An example of it is, "I have mentioned several times that I do not want a drink tonight, and yet you keep pressuring me. Why is it so important to you that I drink?" Regardless of the option selected, clients are taught to monitor their tone of voice and body language when they deliver these messages, since assertive words can be overlooked in the context of an unassertive presentation.

Job skills

A significant "community" for most people is their job environment. Inherent in this is the potential for valuable reinforcement, which may come in the form of stimulating challenges, praise from supervisors, enhanced self-esteem, pleasant social interactions with coworkers, and financial rewards (basic salary and raises). Furthermore, a steady job also competes with drinking and serves as a deterrent as a result of the structure it introduces into a day.

There are three general components to CRA's job counseling program: getting a job, keeping a job, and enhancing job satisfaction. *The Job Club Counselor's Manual* (Azrin & Besalel, 1980) provides the framework for the training of unemployed clients. It offers direction in developing a résumé, completing job applications, and generating and tracking job leads. Behavioral rehearsal is emphasized for both the initial telephone contacts and the actual interviews. Comprehensive monitoring of job-seeking behaviors is built into the process, since this allows us to make behavioral contracts with clients and to reinforce signs of progress. Finally, new job prospects are always considered in terms of their relative risk for promoting drinking.

Obtaining employment is often relatively easy for clients; the difficult part is keeping the job. Consequently energy is devoted to discussing the factors that have contributed to the client being fired or quitting in the past. Many of these may be alcohol or drug related, but others may be due to other factors, such as anger management difficulties or depression. For instances in which the problem is not simply related to substance abuse, either communication skills or problem-solving training might be useful.

The final component of CRA's job program involves an often over-looked topic: enhancing job satisfaction. But again, since CRA works to enhance the level of satisfaction in all nondrinking areas of a person's life, it is important to monitor job satisfaction so that it can be addressed if necessary. The Happiness Scale inquires about job satisfaction, and conse-quently it provides an avenue for determining the extent to which the client generally finds his or her job reinforcing. Reports of significant job dissat-isfaction are explored in depth, and often a solution is attempted through a problem-solving intervention.

Social / recreational counseling

Given that CRA's goal is to make an individual's nondrinking activities as reinforcing as his or her drinking activities, considerable attention must be paid to the client's social life. Unfortunately, many therapists incorrectly assume that individuals will know how to enjoy their free time even if alcohol is no longer a part of it, and consequently they devote little energy to the topic. But it is important to realize that by the time a client enters treatment, it is fairly common for him or her to be enmeshed in a "drinking culture" in which friendships and recreational activities revolve around drinking. Since continued contact with such an environment places the client at risk for relapse, it is critical to explore the idea of spending time with nondrinking friends, and developing more nondrinking pleasurable activities.

Once the need for identifying new nondrinking activities and friends is recognized, many clients require assistance and encouragement before they make any changes in their social life. This may entail guidance in generating lists of options, or completing additional functional analyses for nondrinking behaviors. Importantly, we never assume that a client will follow through and actually try a new activity simply because one has been identified. Instead we determine if there are any obstacles that might interfere with participation, and, if so, problem-solving is utilized. We also rely on a technique called Systematic Encouragement (Sisson & Mallams, 1981) to maximize the chances of the client actually sampling the new activity. The three components of this technique include:

1. Assume that the client probably will have trouble making the first contact on his or her own. Use role-plays to practise phone calls to the organization. After adequate rehearsal and feedback, have the client place the actual call during the session.
2. Locate a contact person for the activity, if possible, and have the client call this individual prior to the event. There is a greater likelihood that the client will attend the activity if arrangements have been made to have a contact person watching for him or her at the event.
3. Be sure to review the experience with the client at the next session to determine whether the activity was sufficiently enjoyable that he or she plans on attending again. Introduce problem-solving to address any difficulties that arose, or select a new activity and repeat the procedure.

If the CRA program is being used to treat a sizeable number of individuals, one might consider organizing a social club similar to the one used in several studies (Mallams et al., 1982; Smith, Meyers & Delaney, 1998). The objective of this club is to show that alcohol-free social activities can be enjoyable, and to provide an event that competes with drinking during high-risk times (e.g., Friday and Saturday nights). Depending on resources and the volume of clients, a clinic could host a "social club" by providing such activities as free video showings, card games, TV sporting events, support meetings, and refreshments.

CRA relationship therapy

It is probably safe to assume that if a problem drinker is living with a loved one, then the relationship is strained. Sometimes the problems in the relationship are partly responsible for the initial onset of excessive drinking, as some individuals attempt to escape emotional distress through alcohol. For others, the drinking problem may have been well established already, but the relationship is now suffering because of continuous arguments over the excessive alcohol use, or because the loved one is withdrawing from the drinker and not communicating. The resultant stress may then serve as a cue for even more imbibing. We believe that focusing exclusively on the client's drinking, while ignoring the interpersonal problems the drinking has stemmed from or created, seriously limits the benefits the drinker may derive from treatment. Consequently, partners typically are invited to participate in segments of the client's program.

The goal of CRA relationship therapy is to make the relationship more reinforcing for both individuals (Azrin, Naster & Jones, 1973; Stuart, 1969). It accomplishes this by teaching problem-solving, by working on the couple's communication, and by showing them how to set realistic goals with each other. The problem-solving procedure already introduced is easily applied to couples' work. The modification is that both individuals participate in each step of the procedure once a problem has been raised and defined by one of them. In terms of communication training for the couple, if the client is considering disulfiram use the training will begin here as part of learning the monitor's role. Regardless, the Relationship Happiness Scale, which is the couple's version of the Happiness Scale, is administered next (see Figure 3.7). Each individual independently indicates his or her degree of satisfaction with the *partner* in ten categories: household responsibilities, raising the children, social activities, money management, communication, sex and affection, job/school, emotional support, partner's independence, and general happiness. As with the Happiness Scale, these categories can be altered to fit the couple's specific needs.

We next share with the couple their individual ratings on the Relationship Happiness Scales, and a discussion of their discrepant perceptions of the problems in the relationship naturally follows. Then a category with at least a moderate degree of satisfaction for both individuals is selected to begin the goal-setting exercise. When the Perfect Relationship form is introduced, the client is told that the guidelines for completing it are the same as those learned for the Goals of Counseling form. In other words, the statements should be brief, positive, and specific (measurable terms). However, for the couples' version the goals are stated for one's *partner*. Each person takes a turn in formulating and then presenting to the loved one a request for some specific type of behavior change. We assist with modifying the wording in accordance with the guidelines.

For example, assume a couple is working on the social activities category, and the wife of the drinker agrees to go first. She begins by stating, "I want him to turn the TV off once in a while and offer to go out to eat, or to a movie, or even just to do errands with me." We reinforce her for primarily using positive terms as far as stating what she would like to see. We point out that her request probably would be received more openly if she dropped the initial negative part about turning "the TV off once in a while", and if she narrowed down her somewhat vague request to one

Relationship Happiness Scale

This scale is intended to estimate your current happiness with your relationship in each of the ten areas listed below. Ask yourself the following question as you rate each area:

How happy am I today with my partner in this area?

Then circle the number that applies.

Numbers toward the left indicate various degrees of unhappiness, while numbers toward the right reflect various levels of happiness.

In other words, by using the proper number you will be indicating just how happy you are with your partner in that particular relationship area.

Remember: You are indicating your current happiness, that is, how you feel today. Also, try not to let your feelings in one area influence the ratings in another area.

	Completely unhappy						Completely happy			
Household responsibilities	1	2	3	4	5	6	7	8	9	10
Raising the children	1	2	3	4	5	6	7	8	9	10
Social activities	1	2	3	4	5	6	7	8	9	10
Money management	1	2	3	4	5	6	7	8	9	10
Communication	1	2	3	4	5	6	7	8	9	10
Sex and affection	1	2	3	4	5	6	7	8	9	10
Job or school	1	2	3	4	5	6	7	8	9	10
Emotional support	1	2	3	4	5	6	7	8	9	10
Partner's independence	1	2	3	4	5	6	7	8	9	10
General happiness	1	2	3	4	5	6	7	8	9	10

Name:_____   Date:_____

Figure 3.7 Relationship Happiness Scale. From *Clinical guide to alcohol treatment: the Community Reinforcement Approach* by R. J. Meyers & J. E. Smith, 1995, p. 171. Copyright 1995 by Guilford Press, New York. Adapted with permission.

specific thing; perhaps even to one specific evening. Also, we suggest that she should first focus on adding activities that are most apt to be experienced as pleasurable and truly social in nature, since they are more likely to be repeated. In other words, the errands could be addressed later under the "household responsibilities" category. Eventually the wife writes on the Perfect Relationship form something similar to, "I would like him to agree to go out to dinner every Friday or Saturday night." The husband is then given his turn to make a request. Assume he states, "I want her to learn to play poker so we can play cards with some friends of mine now and then." We first discuss with the couple the importance of selecting nondrinking social environments. If this does not appear to be a problem, the husband is coached to take this brief, positive statement and make it more specific, "I want her to sit down with me one night a week for about an hour so that I can show her how to play poker." Sometimes negotiation is required before both parties are willing to try complying with the request in the upcoming week. Depending on the couple, an additional request may be practised, or the formulation of it may be given as an assignment (see Figure 3.8 for a page from a partially completed Perfect Relationship Form for the wife in this couple).

Communication skills training follows naturally from the Perfect Relationship exercise, as it builds on the three basic rules and adds the four that had been previously introduced to the client in an individual session: label your feelings, make an understanding statement, accept partial responsibility, and offer to help. The last four guidelines are presented as "advanced" communication skills. A good starting point is to take the statements written on the Perfect Relationship form, as these can be modified and then practised verbally. For example, the wife works on her request about going out to dinner. Eventually her communication approximates, "I would like you to go out to dinner with me every Friday or Saturday night. I know that you're really tired by the end of the week and you'd rather stay home (understanding statement), and it probably doesn't help to have me pressuring you to take me out (partial responsibility). I do feel bad though, when you seem to prefer to watch TV instead of talking to me over dinner (feelings). Maybe it would help if I made a point of either making or ordering us a nice dinner for home for the weekend night that we don't go out (offer to help)." We spend time discussing the different feelings evoked by the polished communications as opposed to the rough initial attempts. The fact that each individual is more likely to have a request honored when it follows most of these guidelines is highlighted. As

Perfect Relationship

Under each area listed below, write down the activities that would represent an ideal relationship.
Be brief, be positive, and state in a specific and measurable way what you would like to see occur.

1. In household responsibilities I would like my partner to:

    1.   *Rinse off his dishes and put them in the dishwasher each evening as he gets up from the table.*

    2. _____

    3. _____

    4. _____

    5. _____

2. In raising the children I would like my partner to:

    1.   *Give the children their baths on Tuesday and Thursday nights (by 7:30).*

    2.   *Take little Nickie on about a 20- to 30-minute bike ride with him once each weekend.*

    3. _____

    4. _____

    5. _____

3. In social activities I would like my partner to:

    1.   *Agree to go out to dinner every Friday or Saturday night.*

    2. _____

    3. _____

    4. _____

    5. _____

Figure 3.8 Perfect Relationship. Sample of completed form.

was the case with the individual client, the couple is also given encouragement to try to add even just a few of these components of a good
conversation, since the improvement will still be marked (see Smith &
Meyers, 1995, for additional examples).

Another segment of CRA relationship therapy revolves around the
Daily Reminder To Be Nice form (see Figure 3.9). In the beginning stages
of couples therapy, most individuals sadly report that they no longer
engage in any of the small, pleasant interactions that used to show how
much they cared about each other. We explain that one goal is to strive for
a relationship that is again tipped in the direction of favoring loving,
enjoyable interactions over unpleasant ones. In order to "jump start" this
process, the Daily Reminder To Be Nice form is given to each individual.
This single-page form simply lists a variety of small, positive behaviors
that one individual can do for another, and leaves room for tracking the
frequency of engaging in these behaviors throughout the week. Although
the categories certainly may be modified to suit a particular couple, the
ones used on the form include:

1. Did you express appreciation to your partner today?
2. Did you compliment your partner today?
3. Did you give your partner any pleasant surprises today?
4. Did you express visible affection to your partner today?
5. Did you spend some time devoting your complete attention to pleasant
   conversation with your partner today?
6. Did you *initiate* a pleasant conversation today?
7. Did you make any offer to help before being asked today?

Not surprisingly, some individuals feel resentful about having to do something pleasant for the drinking partner at the early stages of therapy. We
acknowledge and discuss these feelings. At the same time, the couple is
informed that this is the first step toward making many aspects of their
relationship enjoyable again. Consequently, they are asked to make a
commitment to doing at least one of these behaviors every day. We review
their forms in the next session, and have them verbalize what it felt like to
have their loved one doing pleasant things for them. In short, if a relationship starts to feel supportive and reinforcing for both individuals, then the
chances are greater that it will be able to regularly reinforce a nondrinking
lifestyle.

Daily Reminder To Be Nice

Name: _____

Date:							
Did you express appreciation to your partner today?							
Did you compliment your partner today?							
Did you give your partner any pleasant surprises today?							
Did you express visible affection to your partner today?							
Did you spend some time devoting your complete attention to pleasant conversation with your partner today?							
Did you *initiate* a pleasant conversation today?							
Did you make any offer to help before being asked today?							

Figure 3.9 Daily Reminder To Be Nice form. From *Clinical guide to alcohol treatment: the Community Reinforcement Approach* by R. J. Meyers & J. E. Smith, 1995, p. 179. Copyright 1995 Guilford Press, New York. Adapted with permisssion.

CRA's relapse prevention

Relapse prevention technically begins with the first CRA session, since the CRA Functional Analysis For Drinking Behavior Chart outlines the triggers for alcohol use and identifies high-risk situations. This is followed up with plans to develop behaviors and skills that compete with the drinking. In the event that a lapse occurs, a separate CRA Functional Analysis For Drinking Behavior (Relapse Version) Chart is available. Modeled after the initial assessment version, the relapse chart simply focuses on the one episode and the specific context in which it occurred. Once the context for the lapse is established, the relevant issues are addressed typically by problem-solving or additional skills training.

We also discuss relapse prevention in terms of an Early Warning System. The behavioral chain of events that result in a drinking episode are diagramed, and the client is asked to identify the sequence of warning signals early in the process. For example, assume a client said that he drank several bottles of beer at a friend's house when he only really intended to stop by to talk for a few minutes because he was feeling upset. In recreating the scenario, the client comes to understand that there were actually several warning signals along the way:

1. Feeling agitated and disappointed because the long-awaited fishing trip was canceled at the last minute.
2. Hopping in the car and heading over to a friend's house; one who always has alcohol available.
3. Heading into the friend's kitchen, where innumerable drinking episodes have occurred in the past.
4. Watching his friend head for the refrigerator before they even sit down.
5. Seeing his friend pull out two cold beers and put them on the counter while he looks for a bottle opener.
6. Seeing his friend coming toward him with two open bottles of beer, and hearing him say, "One drink won't hurt."
7. Saying to himself, "I deserve a break now and then" while taking the bottle from his friend and putting it up to his mouth.
8. Seeing his friend hop up and reach into the refrigerator again before they have even finished their first beers.

We remind the client that a number of old drinking triggers could have served as early warning signals: feeling agitated and disappointed, seeking the company of a former drinking buddy who still drinks heavily, going into a setting associated with excessive drinking, being handed a drink with the assurance that one will not be a problem, and feeling sorry for himself. The next step entails formulating a nondrinking plan that starts with the first of the early warning signals and deals with his agitated and disappointed feelings.

General comments

As with all behavioral programs, CRA is only as good as the therapists who administer it. Consequently, if a therapist does not possess good basic clinical skills, the program will be limited. Furthermore, enthusiastic therapists sometimes become fully committed to using the various CRA techniques, but in the process they lose sight of the overall purpose: to help make the person's nondrinking lifestyle as reinforcing as his or her drinking lifestyle. In order to do this one must be constantly aware of the client's reinforcers in all areas of his or her "community", including family, job, and social activities. Having access to these reinforcers on a regular basis is critical in terms of effecting and maintaining change.

4

A Comparison of CRA and Traditional Approaches

WILLIAM R. MILLER, ROBERT J. MEYERS AND
J. SCOTT TONIGAN

The degree of methodological control in Azrin's early studies (reviewed in Chapter 2) and the surprisingly large treatment effects that were obtained established the Community Reinforcement Approach (CRA) as one of the more promising interventions for alcohol problems. The treatment procedures were reasonably well specified, the main effects of intervention were robust, and the largest specific impact was found among less socially stable (e.g., unmarried) clients who would generally be regarded as having a poorer prognosis. On the basis of the Azrin studies alone, several structured reviews of the treatment-outcome literature classified CRA among methods having the strongest empirical evidence of efficacy (e.g., Finney & Monahan, 1996; Holder et al.,1991; Miller et al., 1995).

Addressing limitations of the early studies

Nevertheless, there were important methodological limitations in the early CRA studies, most of which were conducted more than 25 years ago. As we launched a new line of research on CRA, we sought to address these limitations:

- Sample sizes had been quite small.
- CRA had not been tested outside the rural Illinois setting in which it had been developed, and replication was needed with a more heterogeneous population.
- Follow-up had been limited to 6 months in the outpatient trial (Azrin et al., 1982), and a longer course of follow-up was clearly desirable.
- Outcome measurement relied entirely on client self-report.
- The outpatient study had also used the same behavior therapists to conduct both traditional and CRA treatments. This introduced a

potentially serious confound in that these counselors viewed the two treatments quite differently, being enthusiastic about CRA and skeptical about the efficacy of a "traditional" approach. A fairer test of traditional treatment procedures would be to evaluate them in their usual context: service delivery within an ongoing treatment system, where treatments are provided by counselors who are committed to their approach.

- The "traditional" treatment with which CRA was compared had not been well specified. It would be useful to specify more clearly the content of the comparison treatment.
- Follow-up interviews in Azrin's studies were conducted by treatment personnel who were aware of group assignment, and independent follow-up assessment would be highly desirable.
- Finally, Azrin's full "improved" CRA had never been tested without its disulfiram component, which may not be an essential element. The original, less elaborate CRA program (Hunt & Azrin, 1973) had not included disulfiram, but nevertheless was found to be highly effective. Given uncertainty about the efficacy and safety of this medication (Miller & Hester, 1986), the necessary and/or sufficient role of disulfiram within CRA needed to be addressed.

A replication and extension

With these methodological issues in mind, we designed an independent replication and extension of the Illinois research, referred to hereafter as the CASAA study. The design was a randomized clinical trial building on Azrin's work. With a larger sample of clients, we tested CRA in an ongoing public outpatient treatment program – the University of New Mexico Center on Alcoholism, Substance Abuse, and Addictions (CASAA), the largest public provider of addiction treatment services in New Mexico. The study was designed specifically to answer these seven questions:

1. Is CRA superior to traditional treatment procedures, and, if so, how large is its specific effect? We were particularly interested in whether we could replicate the large treatment effect reported by Azrin and his colleagues in the Illinois studies.
2. Does the disulfiram-compliance component of CRA significantly improve treatment outcomes relative to a standard disulfiram administration procedure? Azrin had introduced a novel procedure to enhance compliance with disulfiram by training a significant other to monitor

and facilitate medication adherence. How much would this contribute to ordinary disulfiram prescription procedures used in traditional treatment?

3. Does the full CRA yield significantly greater improvement than traditional treatment plus a disulfiram-compliance program, either for the total population or for a definable subgroup? This question is the inverse of number 2: how much does CRA improve outcome compared to more traditional treatments including disulfiram? Azrin had reported that, with married clients, the addition of a disulfiram-compliance procedure to traditional treatment yielded the same magnitude of change as the full CRA package, whereas for unmarried clients the full CRA was substantially better (Azrin et al., 1982).

4. To what extent is the effectiveness of CRA compromised when disulfiram is not included, in a population otherwise able and willing to take it? We wanted to address the unanswered question of how important disulfiram is to the effectiveness of the "improved" CRA treatment method. To do so, it was important to start with clients who were willing and able to take disulfiram, and randomize them to receive or not receive it.

5. Among clients for whom disulfiram is contraindicated or refused, does CRA (without disulfiram) significantly improve treatment outcomes, relative to traditional treatment procedures? Another unanswered question, this pertained to clients who were ineligible or unwilling to take disulfiram. Such clients had been excluded from earlier trials, and we wanted to know whether CRA would benefit them.

6. How enduring are the effects of the specific interventions under study? Finally, we were interested in following clients for a longer period of time than the 3–6 months covered in prior studies. Would observed treatment effects endure over the course of one to two years?

7. We also had an ancillary interest in client–treatment matching. For whom does CRA yield the greatest benefit, relative to traditional treatment procedures? Is there an identifiable subgroup of clients for whom CRA (or traditional) treatment is differentially beneficial? Very large samples are required to provide statistical power to test interaction effects (e.g., Project MATCH Research Group, 1997), so this was regarded as an exploratory issue in the present study.

Because we sought to replicate Azrin's studies, we used similar treatment procedures and outcome measures. To answer questions that had not been addressed in the Illinois studies, we added groups that received CRA without disulfiram. A range of pretreatment characteristics was assessed to search for optimal pretreatment matching strategies, in addition to replicating Azrin's finding of differential efficacy based on marital status. Clients for whom disulfiram was inappropriate were not excluded from the study, but were entered into a separate randomized trial to test the efficacy of CRA without disulfiram. Follow-up by interviewers unaware of group assignment was extended for a period of two years. Traditional treatment procedures were administered by highly experienced CASAA counselors who were committed to a disease model and a 12-step approach. Likewise, CRA procedures were delivered by experienced CASAA counselors, whose training and orientation were consistent with this behavioral approach. Treatment drop-outs were followed, and the study sample was culturally diverse. A range of outcome measures was included to document drinking, alcohol-related problems and dependence, psychological adjustment, employment, and institutionalization.

Design of the CASAA study

We replicated Azrin's outpatient study (Azrin et al., 1982) by reproducing the same three treatment conditions: (1) traditional treatment alone, (2) traditional treatment plus disulfiram compliance, and (3) full CRA. To these we added another group (4), who received CRA without disulfiram, in order to determine the extent to which disulfiram contributes to the overall effectiveness of the CRA. As in Azrin's study, this comparison necessitated that all clients be willing and medically eligible to take disulfiram.

Because disulfiram eligibility limits the population to be treated, perhaps selecting better prognosis cases, we added another dimension to the proposed design. All clients who were ineligible for the above trial, by virtue of their refusal of or contraindications to disulfiram, were assigned at random to one of two groups: (5) traditional treatment, or (6) CRA without disulfiram (reproducing Groups 1 and 4 from the disulfiram-eligible arm of the study). This provision assessed the differential effectiveness of CRA within a disulfiram-ineligible population. The design is shown in Table 4.1.

Sample inclusion criteria

The trial sample was drawn from the CASAA's regular clinical population. Clients were offered the opportunity to participate in the study when presenting for initial evaluation for treatment services. Potential

Table 4.1. *Design of the CASAA study*

Disulfiram eligible (Groups 1–4)				Disulfiram ineligible (Groups 5, 6)	
Traditional treatment	Traditional treatment	CRA treatment	CRA treatment	Traditional treatment	CRA treatment
Group 1 Disulfiram optional	Group 2 Disulfiram compliance	Group 3 Disulfiram compliance	Group 4 No disulfiram	Group 5 No disulfiram	Group 6 No disulfiram

participants were all CASAA clients who: (1) met problem-ascertainment criteria (see below), (2) showed no obvious impediment to comprehending assessment and treatment (e.g., acute psychosis or organic brain syndrome, inability to read English at 8th grade level), (3) resided within Bernalillo County (population 500,000), and (4) consented to participate in the study. Clients seeking CASAA services during the 16-month enrollment period were screened by project staff to determine eligibility on these criteria. Those who were eligible were given a full disclosure of study conditions, and reviewed and signed a statement of informed consent in accord with procedures approved by the University of New Mexico School of Medicine Institutional Review Board for human research.

Exclusion criteria

Screening next determined the individual's medical eligibility for and willingness to take disulfiram. Based on this determination by Dr P. J. Abbott, the client was assigned to either the disulfiram-eligible or the disulfiram-ineligible randomized trial (see Table 4.1). Standard contraindications for disulfiram were: (1) recent myocardial infarction or other significant cardiovascular pathology, especially cardiac conduction problems; (2) pregnancy; (3) significant elevation of liver enzymes (gamma glutamyl transpeptidase, GGTP, >100 U/l), or (4) insulin-dependent diabetes mellitus. As further precautions: (5) clients with GGTP values between 60 and 100 U/l were scheduled for repeated serum GGTP assays at each follow-up point during disulfiram administration, to ensure against continued elevation; (6) clients currently maintained on anticonvulsant medications were monitored regularly for medication level, to ensure against hazardous elevation due to disulfiram administration; and (7) a final screening step, also supervised by Dr P. J. Abbott and intended to increase sample homogeneity, ruled out clients with affective disorders of sufficient severity to require psychiatric medication during the course of treatment.

Pretreatment assessment

A standard pretreatment assessment battery was administered to all participants. The assessment procedures that are standard components of intake evaluation at CASAA were administered as usual by clinical personnel. Special pretreatment assessment procedures unique to this study were administered by research staff. All pretreatment assessment was conducted prior to the randomization to treatment conditions.

Breath test

Prior to pretreatment assessment (and every assessment and treatment session), a breath alcohol test was administered. The presence of any alcohol (>0.01 g%) was recorded, and the session rescheduled. This was done to ensure sobriety at the time of informed consent, to promote greater accuracy of self-report and testing results, and to facilitate comprehension of treatment.

Problem ascertainment

The first level of pretreatment assessment served to establish the presence of alcohol problems. To be admitted to the study, all clients were required to score within the symptomatic range on at least two of the following four measures:

1. *The Addiction Severity Index* (McLellan et al., 1980). The pertinent scale for this purpose was the alcohol scale. A cut-score of 5 was used to define alcohol problems.
2. *The DSM-III-R Criteria for Alcohol Dependence Syndrome.* A minimum of four out of nine dependence symptoms were required to meet this criterion, according to the *Diagnostic and statistical manual of mental disorders* (American Psychiatric Association, 1980).
3. *The Alcohol Use Inventory* (Horn, Wanberg & Foster, 1987). As a psychometric measure of alcohol problems and dependence, we used the D-1 (Alcoholic Deterioration) factor of the Alcohol Use Inventory

(Revised). A minimum score of 10 (third decile or above, relative to norms for clients in treatment for alcohol problems) was required to meet this criterion.

4. *Gamma glutamyl transpeptidase (GGTP)*. As a biomedical indicator, we used GGTP elevation as a marker of excessive alcohol consumption and long-term risk for alcohol-related impairment (Kristenson et al., 1983; Reyes & Miller, 1980). An elevation in excess of our laboratory normal range (> 60 U/l) was counted as meeting the criterion on this measure.

Drinking measures

The Brief Drinker Profile (Miller & Marlatt, 1987), a shortened version of the Comprehensive Drinker Profile (Miller & Marlatt, 1984), was used as a structured research intake interview. It provides pretreatment information including demographics and quantitative indices of alcohol consumption, family history of alcoholism, alcohol-related life problems, alcohol dependence, other drug use, and treatment motivation. Each participant was also asked to provide the names and telephone numbers of up to three significant others who could serve as locators and collateral information sources. These collaterals were interviewed using the Collateral Interview Form, which parallels content of the Brief Drinker Profile (Miller, Crawford & Taylor, 1979; Miller & Marlatt, 1987). For all these interviews, drinking data were converted into the total number of standard drinks (0.5 oz or 15 ml of absolute ethanol; Miller, Heather & Hall, 1991) consumed per week. We also estimated peak weekly blood alcohol concentration (BAC) by computer projection (Markham, Miller & Arciniega, 1993) based on gender, body mass, volume and spacing of alcohol consumption.

Other measures

The Symptom Checklist (SCL-90-R) was completed by each client as an indicator of psychological status (Derogatis, 1983; Derogatis & Melisaratos, 1983; Derogatis, Rickels & Rock, 1976). Baseline depressive symptoms were assessed via the Hamilton (1960) Rating Scale for depression. A serum sample was drawn and assayed to yield a blood chemistry panel. An early version of the Stages of Change Readiness and Treatment Eagerness Scale (SOCRATES; Miller & Tonigan, 1996) was also included in the pretreatment assessment battery as a motivational measure, along with the University of Rhode Island Change Assessment (URICA; DiClemente & Hughes, 1990). We measured clients' satisfaction with their treatment and therapist using a specially designed questionnaire with Likert-type rating scales. Four items focused on treatment satisfaction, and five additional items rated specific therapist qualities of understanding, ability to listen, interest in the client, overall competence, and the extent to which the client liked the assigned therapist.

Disulfiram compliance

Within the disulfiram-eligible population, breath tests were planned to verify disulfiram compliance, following the procedures of Kraml (1973) to detect carbon disulfide. Rychtarik et al. (1983) had reported the carbon disulfide breath test to be a sensitive indicator of disulfiram compliance. A Wright respirometer was used, and the test chemicals were prepared by a faculty member of the University of New Mexico Department of Pharmacology, according to instructions provided by Rychtarik et al. The tests were administered by a registered research nurse and several research assistants. From the beginning, there were substantial discrepancies between client self-reports of disulfiram compliance and breath test results. When negative test results were obtained for several clients at follow-up who had been directly observed by CASAA staff to be taking liquid disulfiram on a daily basis, we administered breath tests to additional volunteers, known to be taking daily disulfiram. We found that many of these tests were negative, and that the same subjects produced varying results from one day to the next. Several new batches of test solution were prepared after confirming proper procedures with Rychtarik et al. Again, known positive cases often yielded negative test results. Consequently, part way through the trial, we abandoned the disulfiram breath test procedure as unreliable in our hands.

Group assignment

Stratified random group assignment was accomplished in the following manner. Slips of paper were marked for each treatment group in the design, and these were mixed together within urns for disulfiram-eligible (Groups 1–4, $n=160$) and disulfiram-ineligible (Groups 5 and 6, $n=80$) clients. Slips were then drawn one at a time from the urns, designating the sequence of assignment of clients to groups. These slips were sealed in opaque envelopes and numbered in sequence, corresponding to the order in which they had been drawn. This resulted in two sets of group-assignment envelopes, one for each arm of the study, designed to produce groups of equal size ($n=40$).

Marital status was a key predictor of outcomes in Azrin's outpatient study of CRA (Azrin et al., 1982). To ensure an adequate representation of married clients (26% of CASAA's clients were married and living with their partners) and approximate a balance of marital status across groups, the final one-third of envelopes in each assignment sequence was reserved for married or cohabiting clients. The intent was to guarantee a minimum of one-third married clients within each group. The assignment envelope for each client was therefore drawn from among the envelopes for married or single individuals, depending upon the client's marital status at intake. The planned procedure was to stop accepting unmarried clients into the trial if two-thirds (26 per group) were recruited before one-third (14 per group) married clients had been entered. In fact, over one-third of recruited clients were married, making it unnecessary to close recruitment of unmarried clients.

A quandary was posed by clients who consented (prior to randomization) to take disulfiram, but then refused after entering a treatment group that required the medication, thus rendering them inappropriate for the disulfiram-eligible arm of the study (in that refusal to take disulfiram was an exclusion criterion for this arm). There were nine such refusals in Group 2 (traditional) and one in Group 3 (CRA). (Groups 1, 4, 5, and 6 were not required to take disulfiram as part of their treatment.) Because the disulfiram-compliance procedure was a distinguishing element of Groups 2 and 3, and of central interest in experimental analyses, we removed these cases (usually during the first two sessions) from their original treatment condition and replaced them with new cases. Refusals from Group 2 were reassigned to the treatment received by corresponding Group 5, and the refusal from Group 3 was reassigned to the same treatment received by Group 6. New numbers were assigned from the envelopes for Groups 5 and 6, but these cases were not included in the final analyses for these groups. Ten additional cases were then assigned to the disulfiram-ineligible arm of the study to provide the full n of 80. This retained true randomization for the compared groups, but the procedure led to an unforeseen consequence. Because the order of assignment had been determined for the full complement of cases in one drawing, the ten additional clients were assigned to Groups 5 or 6 by coin toss. This turned out to be an unfortunate choice, because we did not anticipate the uneven rates of migrations into Groups 5 and 6 from Groups 2 and 3, respectively. Our resulting cell sizes in Groups 5 and 6 (excluding refusals from Groups 2 and 3) were thus uneven: 34 and 46, respectively.

Treatment conditions

Treatment fees ordinarily charged on a sliding scale to CASAA clients were waived for all study participants. The target number of treatment sessions in all conditions was 12. The six treatment conditions were:

Group 1: traditional treatment

Treatment of clients in this condition was designed to mirror the standard practices of CASAA counselors at the time the study was initiated (in 1988), operating within what Brickman and colleagues (1982) have characterized as a compensatory model. Two nongraduate counselors, with 15 and 18 years respectively of experience in treating alcoholism and who practised similar disease-oriented counseling approaches, were chosen for this group. A standard core of procedures was specified for all clients in this condition, who were: (1) immediately encouraged to attend meetings of Alcoholics Anonymous (AA), given a schedule of local meetings, and told which meetings might be most appropriate; (2) familiarized with AA literature and the 12–step approach; (3) taught about AA sponsorship and encouraged to obtain an AA sponsor; (4) given an explanation of Jellinek's and Keller's (1952) description of gamma alcoholism as a progressive disease, using the familiar U-shaped curve of deterioration and recovery derived from Jellinek's stages; (5) shown the Father Martin (no date) film, "*Chalk Talk*"; and (6) asked to attend an evening recovery group held at CASAA, facilitated by one of the two therapists and emphasizing a disease model and AA principles. Individual sessions with the counselor were normally scheduled once weekly in this and all treatment groups, with allowance for more frequent sessions if deemed necessary by the counselor. The approach was conceptually similar to the 12-step facilitation treatment later developed and tested in Project MATCH (Nowinski, Baker & Carroll, 1994).

In accord with traditional treatment procedures at the time, Group 1 clients were also encouraged to take disulfiram, by attending one

Antabuse® clinic orientation group session offered twice weekly by a staff psychologist, a physician's assistant, or a counselor. Following this orientation, clients could begin receiving regular doses (500 mg) of disulfiram free of charge. Prescriptions were renewed monthly and reviewed by medical staff, and were normally held and dispensed at CASAA's pharmacy. A Licensed Practical Nurse provided the disulfiram either mixed in a small cup of Kool-Aid® or in pill form taken with water. (The form of administration was decided by the client in consultation with his or her counselor.) During weekends, holiday periods, and any other times when CASAA was closed or clients were to be out of town, take-home doses of disulfiram were given.

Group 2: traditional treatment plus disulfiram-compliance group

Clients assigned to Group 2 received the same traditional treatment components as those in Group 1. In addition, they were given only the disulfiram-compliance procedure of the CRA (Sisson & Azrin, 1986), for which they were asked to bring a spouse or significant other with them to their first session. The spouse or significant other was instructed to serve as a monitor for the client's regular taking of disulfiram. It was explained that the monitor's purpose was only to provide support, and that they were not to have a "watchdog" or "police" role. A 1-month supply of disulfiram tablets was provided, with the prescription specifying that the client should take one 250-mg tablet daily. The daily procedure was for the monitor to dissolve a disulfiram tablet in a glass of water or juice, and then offer it to the client. The monitor was also coached to praise the client for making such a commitment to staying sober. Daily doses of disulfiram were specifically to be accompanied by this type of praise, expression of the monitor's positive feelings, and offers to help in any way. The monitor was cautioned not to argue with or react negatively to the client during this time. If the client refused the disulfiram, the monitor was instructed to be firm and to try to persuade him or her to take it by using positive communication skills, understanding, and empathic statements (Azrin, Naster & Jones, 1973). If the client still refused to take disulfiram for 2 days in a row, the monitor was instructed to call the counselor for advice.

Because Group 2 required this specific CRA counseling procedure, which departed from the ordinary practices of traditional counselors, treatment in Group 2 was provided by one of four CRA counselors. This replicated the work of Azrin et al. (1982), who added their disulfiram-compliance intervention to a traditional treatment program offered by the same counselors who delivered CRA treatment.

Group 3: CRA with disulfiram compliance

Group 3 received the same disulfiram-compliance intervention as Group 2, but rather than being given traditional treatment they received the full CRA program, as described by Azrin (1976; Azrin et al., 1982). The CRA protocol consisted of a series of four to six individual one-hour sessions, followed by monthly check-in sessions for several months. The number of sessions was determined jointly by the counselor and client, judging from the client's progress and perceived need for additional contact. (This was preferred to a fixed duration of treatment, because it more nearly approximates clinical practice.) The full CRA program included:

1. *Sobriety sampling.* The client's motivational reasons for sobriety were reviewed, and the client was encouraged to "sample" sobriety by trying a negotiated period of abstinence.
2. *Disulfiram compliance.* To assist in sobriety, clients were encouraged to use disulfiram, with the monitoring program described for Group 2.
3. *Functional analysis.* A detailed functional analysis of high-risk situations was conducted for each client, examining the relationships between drinking behavior and environmental antecedents and consequences.
4. *Problem-solving training.* Clients were given training in general problem-solving skills, with strategies and behavioral rehearsal directed toward their individual problem situations.
5. *Social skill training.* Clients were taught basic strategies for effective social communication, such as making understanding (empathic) statements, accepting partial responsibility for interpersonal difficulties, and offering to help (Azrin et al., 1982; Sisson & Azrin, 1986).
6. *Social counseling.* Clients were encouraged and assisted to schedule rewarding activities, develop hobbies or recreational pursuits, take advantage of community resources, and seek the company of nondrinking companions and friends to support their sobriety. This was emphasized particularly for clients who were socially isolated, or who needed social activities to compete with and replace drinking time.
7. *Mood monitoring.* Clients were taught to monitor mood on a daily basis, as an early warning system to detect signs of impending relapse. The client was instructed, on observing warning signs, to resume contact with the counselor. For married clients, the spouse was also encouraged to monitor the client's mood for warning signs, and to initiate counselor contact in problem situations.

Beyond these core elements designed for all clients, procedures from a CRA menu were chosen by the counselor to meet each client's needs:

8. *Job-finding counseling.* Clients who were unemployed were encouraged to attend a job-finding club offered at CASAA every weekday morning. The club was operated by a specially trained counselor, whose half-time responsibility was operation of the job-counseling program. Procedures for the job club have been fully detailed by Azrin and Besalel (1980). Copies of the book *Finding a job* (Azrin & Besalel, 1982) were given to participants.

9. *Behavioral marital therapy.* For clients experiencing problems within a marital or other intimate relationship, reciprocity counseling (Azrin, Naster & Jones, 1973) was provided, focused on increasing positive communication and exchange of reinforcement within the relationship.

10. *Reinforcer access counseling.* Isolated clients were encouraged and given practical assistance in obtaining access to common sources of information and reinforcement: a radio or television, newspaper and magazines, a driver's license, a telephone, etc.

11. *Relaxation training.* For clients suffering from anxiety problems, progressive deep muscle relaxation training was offered (Rosen, 1977).

12. *Drink refusal.* For clients who had difficulty in refusing unwanted drinks, assertiveness training was provided to increase their ability to resist. Both instruction and practice were included.

Group 4: CRA without disulfiram

Clients assigned to Group 4 received the same CRA as described for Group 3, except that disulfiram was not prescribed or encouraged.

Group 5: traditional treatment without disulfiram

Groups 5 and 6 were the assignment options for disulfiram-ineligible clients. Treatment given to Group 5 was identical to that for Group 1, and delivered by the same traditional counselors, except that disulfiram was not prescribed or encouraged.

Group 6: CRA without disulfiram

The treatment given to Group 6 was identical to that described above for Group 4.

Quality control

A 6-month period was devoted to the development of a consistent set of CRA procedures and a therapist manual (later refined and published as Meyers & Smith, 1995), to the initial training of CRA therapists by three members of Azrin's original clinical team, and to supervised practice with nontrial cases. The CRA therapists met weekly with their supervisor (Meyers) to discuss cases and maintain protocol adherence. Because both of the traditional therapists had over 15 years of experience as traditional alcoholism counselors, and none of the procedures included in the final protocol departed from their routine practice, we developed an outline of points and procedures to be covered in treatment rather than a formal manual. No additional training was provided for the traditional treatment condition. These therapists also met weekly with their supervisor, and also with Dr Meyers regarding research protocols. Consistent with standard clinical practice at the time, the treatment sessions were not recorded on audio or videotape.

Attrition from treatment

Once clients had been randomized and attended an initial treatment session, they were considered to be trial subjects and were followed regardless of further compliance. Clients who completed all or part of pretreatment assessment but did not return for their first treatment session were regarded as study drop-outs, were not followed, and were replaced in the randomization sequence.

For purposes of analyses, we also needed a criterion for when clients should be considered as having received a sufficient dose of treatment to be considered as "treated". Clients who attended only one or two treatment sessions, regardless of group assignment, were regarded as treatment drop-outs, but were included in normal follow-up procedures. Clients who attended at least three treatment sessions were regarded as treated, and counted as such in analyses.

Follow-up assessment

Follow-up interviews were planned for 2, 3, 4, 6, 9, 12, 18, and 24 months following treatment intake, using a standard Follow-up Drinker Profile interview protocol (Miller & Marlatt, 1987) to document alcohol consumption, life problems, other drug use, and alcohol-dependence symptoms. Collateral interviews were also conducted at these intervals, obtaining information to parallel self-report data. At 6, 12, and 24 months, the SCL-90-R, the Addiction Severity Index, and the serum chemistry profile were readministered. Follow-up interviewers were uninformed of the clients' group assignment, and cases were rotated among assessors to minimize the effect that treatment group information inadvertently obtained at one interview would have on subsequent follow-up interviews.

If follow-ups were not completed during the target week, persistent efforts were made to contact and interview subjects. Telephone interviews were completed in cases where efforts to conduct an in-person interview were infeasible (moved out of the state) or repeatedly unsuccessful. Home visits were used to obtain follow-up data when telephone interviews could not be completed. The window for a follow-up interview was considered to extend until 1 week before the due date for the next follow-up interview, after which the follow-up was regarded as missed. In such cases, when the client was interviewed at a subsequent follow-up point, the interviewer reconstructed the missing interval (cf. Grant et al., 1997). Following the recommendation of Gorenstein (1985), the more recent interval was used as an anchor period against which previous intervals were compared and reconstructed.

In addition to a review of treatment charts, checks on services delivered were completed in two ways. At follow-up points immediately following treatment termination, clients were asked (using a questionnaire) to provide two types of information regarding the treatment they had received at CASAA: (1) a report of the setting (individual, group), type (counseling, lecture, disulfiram administration), and amount (number, length) of treatment contacts, to serve as a check against clinical records to verify treatment received; and (2) a rating of the client's satisfaction with treatment received (Attkisson & Zwick, 1982). During the course of treatment, therapists also completed a checklist of procedures delivered, and these were reviewed for compliance during weekly meetings.

In order to increase participation in follow-up interviews, financial incentives were offered for continued contact and completion of assessment. Our initial plan had been to use a lottery incentive system, whereby each subject completing a follow-up interview was eligible for a random drawing to award cash prizes. The proposed ratio was one $100 prize for each 40 subjects at each follow-up point, and one per 30 participants at the most distal follow-ups. We had found in earlier single-visit studies that this procedure provided at least as great an incentive for participation as a modest subject fee paid to every participant, and reduced subject fee costs by more than 70%. Our experience during the present trial, however, reflected a rapid drop-off in the incentive value of the lottery (except for clients who won on early rounds), which increased the difficulty of maintaining high follow-up rates. Consequently we shifted, during the second year of the study, first to an individual subject payment of $10 per interview, and then to $20 per interview, which we found sufficient to motivate participation. Travel costs were occasionally reimbursed for clients residing within New Mexico but outside the Albuquerque metropolitan area at the time of follow-up. Public transportation assistance (bus tokens, taxi) was given as needed for clients to attend assessment sessions.

Project personnel

Administration of the project was overseen by two supervisory staff. Research assistants (University of New Mexico graduate students in clinical psychology) who conducted assessment interviews were trained by the senior author and supervised by a Project Coordinator. During this trial therapists worked on the project on a volunteer basis. There was no money available from the grant to pay supervisors or therapists. No videotapes or audiotapes were utilized for supervisory purposes and no complete manuals were used by either group. Therapist compliance to strict protocol standards was dubious.

All six therapists were CASAA staff, whose duties included the treatment of regular CASAA clients as well as research clients. The two traditional (Groups 1 and 5) therapists both had over 15 years of experience in alcoholism treatment, and neither had university degrees. Three of the four CRA therapists (Groups 2, 3, 4, and 6) held masters degrees or the equivalent, and the more recently hired staff had substantially less (an average of 2 years) clinical experience with alcohol problems.

Data preparation

The raw interview and questionnaire data from the project were subjected to several stages of entry and verification, to ensure accuracy of the data set. First, a data coding sheet was developed to encode variables of interest. Research assistants, in most cases those who had collected the data, completed a first pass of coding the data onto these sheets from the original file. The coding sheets were next double-checked against the original file by a second research assistant, and discrepancies were resolved by the senior author or Project Coordinator. Data were then double-entered from the coding sheets by two technicians, again consulting the original file to resolve questions or apparent inconsistencies.

Each analysis was conducted with all available cases (intent to treat), and a small number of outliers were eliminated prior to each analysis (never more than four per analysis). Statistical outliers were defined as data points lying more than three standard deviations from the mean (Harris, 1985; Tabachnick & Fidell, 1989).

5

Community Reinforcement and Traditional Approaches: Findings of a Controlled Trial

WILLIAM R. MILLER, ROBERT J. MEYERS, J. SCOTT TONIGAN
AND KATHRYN A. GRANT

This chapter contains the primary report of findings from our comparison of the Community Reinforcement (CRA) and traditional approaches, the methodology of which is described in Chapter 4. Our analyses focused on five main topics around which this chapter is organized:

1. Who were the clients we treated?
2. Were the treatments delivered as planned?
3. How well were treatment outcomes documented?
4. Did the compared treatments differ in effectiveness? (Questions 1–6 outlined in Chapter 4.)
5. Were there characteristics of therapists or clients who did particularly well in these treatments? (Question 7 from Chapter 4.)

Sample characteristics

Demographics

As described in Chapter 4, study participants completed a comprehensive assessment at intake that included measurement of numerous demographic characteristics, motivation for change, psychological functioning, drinking history, and current drinking practices. Basic demographic characteristics are presented in Table 5.1 for the total recruited sample ($n = 237$) as well as for the clients who were defined as having received the intended treatment (three or more sessions) versus those clients who dropped out of treatment (two or fewer therapy sessions). As shown, the average client was a male around age 30, who had completed high school but not college. The majority of the sample were Hispanic, and only one in five clients was married at the time of study recruitment. Over 40% of the total sample was unemployed, with an additional 16% reporting only part-time employment.

Table 5.1. *Characteristics of the* total sample, treated cases, *and* drop-outs

Demographic variables	Total sample ($n = 237$)	Treated cases[1] ($n = 192$)	Drop-outs ($n = 45$)	t-test p
Mean age in years	31.17 (7.94)	31.30 (8.19)	30.58 (6.85)	$p < 0.30$
Mean years in education	12.01 (1.98)	11.95 (1.95)	12.29 (2.10)	
Marital status[2]	$n(\%)$	$n(\%)$	$n(\%)$	$\chi^2 p$
Single	110 (46.4%)	94 (49.0%)	16 (35.6%)	$p < 0.09$
Married	51 (21.5%)	37 (19.3%)	14 (31.1%)	
Separated	18 (7.6%)	14 (7.3%)	4 (9.0%)	
Widowed	1 (0.4%)	1 (0.5%)	(0)	
Divorced	57 (24.1%)	46 (24.0%)	11 (5.7%)	
Ethnicity[3]	$n(\%)$	$n(\%)$	$n(\%)$	$\chi^2 p$
Anglo	86 (38.1%)	70 (40.0%)	16 (43.2%)	$p < 0.72$
Hispanic	126 (55.8)	105 (60.0%)	21 (56.8%)	
Native American	9 (4.0%)	6 (3.3%)	3 (7.5%)	
Other	2 (0.8%)	2 (1.1%)	0	
Gender	$n(\%)$	$n(\%)$	$n(\%)$	$\chi^2 p$
Male	196 (82.7%)	163 (84.9%)	33 (73.3%)	$p < 0.08$
Female	41 (17.3%)	29 (15.1%)	12 (26.7%)	
Employment[4]	$n(\%)$	$n(\%)$	$n(\%)$	$\chi^2 p$
Full-time	97 (40.9%)	79 (41.1%)	18 (40.0%)	$p < 0.50$
Part-time	38 (16.0%)	33 (17.2%)	5 (11.1%)	
Unemployed	97 (40.9%)	80 (41.7%)	22 (48.9%)	
Homemaker	5 (2.1%)	4 (2.1%)	1 (2.2%)	
Referral source	$n(\%)$	$n(\%)$	$n(\%)$	$\chi^2 p$
Self-referred	90 (38.8%)	68 (36.4%)	22 (48.9%)	$p < 0.21$
Mental health	20 (8.6%)	17 (9.1%)	3 (6.7%)	
Medical	17 (7.3%)	12 (6.4%)	5 (11.1%)	
Legal	105 (45.3%)	90 (48.1%)	15 (33.3%)	
Drinking pattern	$n(\%)$	$n(\%)$	$n(\%)$	$\chi^2 p$
Episodic only	31 (13.1 %)	29 (15.1%)	2 (4.4%)	$p < 0.09$
Steady	88 (37.1%)	68 (35.4%)	20 (44.4%)	
Both	118 (49.8%)	95 (49.5%)	23 (51.1%)	
Problem severity				
Mean ADS score	16.40 (8.91)	16.50 (8.89)	16.00 (9.09)	$p < 0.74$
Mean DSM signs	9.96 (1.72)	7.01 (1.72)	6.77 (1.72)	$p < 0.41$
Mean MAST	26.82 (10.95)	26.93 (10.82)	26.36 (11.60)	$p < 0.75$
Mean depression	7.57 (6.30)	7.68 (6.47)	7.11 (5.53)	$p < 0.59$
Motivation for change (URICA means)				
Precontemplation	16.47 (5.87)	16.45 (5.87)	16.56 (5.94)	$p < 0.91$
Contemplation	31.47 (4.51)	31.69 (4.50)	30.56 (4.51)	$p < 0.13$
Determination	33.37 (5.68)	33.38 (5.63)	33.32 (5.98)	$p < 0.95$
Action	32.51 (5.28)	32.84 (4.97)	31.13 (6.34)	$p < 0.05$

Table 5.1 (*cont.*)

Demographic variables	Total sample ($n = 237$)	Treated cases ($n = 192$)	Drop-outs ($n = 45$)	t-test p
Drinking and problems				
Years of problem	8.65 (6.65)	8.90 (6.57)	7.58 (6.97)	$p < 0.23$
Alcohol problems	4.62 (3.48)	4.63 (3.40)	4.56 (3.82)	$p < 0.90$
Maximum BAC	0.37 (0.18)	0.37 (0.18)	0.36 (0.18)	$p < 0.92$
Standard drinks	862.7 (786.1)	818.2 (762.1)	1053.1 (864.7)	$p < 0.07$
Drinking days/week	4.51 (2.53)	4.43 (2.57)	4.87 (2.32)	$p < 0.29$
Liver enzymes				
AST (SGOT, U/1)	52.80 (65.13)	51.77 (66.19)	57.13 (61.0)	$p < 0.62$
GGTP (U/1)	124.3 (218.2)	118.7 (197.3)	148.2 (291.6)	$p < 0.42$
Bilirubun	0.63 (0.41)	0.66 (0.44)	0.51 (0.23)	$p < 0.03$
ALT (SGPT, U/1)	61.0 (83.0)	59.1 (85.1)	69.1 (73.9)	$p < 0.47$

[1] Clients attending three or more treatment sessions.
[2] Differential rate examined by χ^2 with married category versus all other categories.
[3] Differential rate examined by χ^2 with Anglo and Hispanic clients only.
[4] Differential rate examined by χ^2 with Homemaker collapsed into unemployed.
ALT, alanine aminotransferase (formerly known as GPT); ADS, Alcohol Dependence Scale; AST, aspartate aminotransferase (formerly known as GOT); BAC, blood alcohol concentration; GGTP, gamma glutamyl transpeptidase; MAST, Michigan Alcoholism Screening Test; SGOT, serum glutamic oxalacetic transaminase; SGPT, serum glutamic pyruvic transaminase; URICA, University of Rhode Island Change Assessment.

Most clients (192, or 81%) remained in treatment long enough (three or more sessions) to have been exposed to the intended approach. A comparison of treated and drop-out cases indicated that there was no significant relationship to any of the demographic variables (Table 5.1).

Drinking variables

Table 5.1 also presents six domains depicting drinking practices and related problems for the recruited sample. About equal proportions of the total sample were self versus legal referrals for alcohol treatment. Most clients had a regular weekly drinking pattern, with just 13% reporting only episodic drinking in the 90 days before treatment. Baseline data reflect the presence of relatively severe alcohol-related problems. Clients met, on average, seven of nine DSM-IIIR symptoms of alcohol dependence (only three required for diagnosis; American Psychiatric Association, 1987), and the average Michigan Alcoholism Screening Test (MAST; Selzer, 1971) (mean = 26.82, SD = 10.95) and Alcohol Dependence Scale scores (mean = 16.40, SD = 8.91) were also consistent with high severity. The average client also showed elevated signs of depression (on the Hamilton Rating Scale), and interviewers tended to rate clients' need for alcohol treatment to be high (on the Addiction Severity Index).

Clients reported an average of 9 years of problem drinking before entering the study. Self-reported amounts of drinking were high for the preceding 90-day period: clients reported a mean of 862.7 standard drinks (0.5 oz or 15 ml ethanol) during the period, which translates into 9.7 drinks per day assuming daily drinking. Clients, however, reported drinking on only 4.5 days per week on average, indicating a mean of 15 standard drinks per drinking day. This is consistent with the computer-projected average peak blood alcohol concentration (BAC) of 370 mg%, and with elevated mean liver enzyme values, particularly gamma glutamyl transpeptidase (GGTP).

Motivation for change

Table 5.1 reflects a relatively high level of motivation for change in drinking behavior, consistent with presentation for treatment. Each of the four scales of the University of Rhode Island Change Assessment (URICA) has a possible range of 8–40 points. Sample means show low precontemplation scores (denial of a problem) and high contemplation, determination, and action scores. The only between-group difference exceeding $p < 0.05$ is that clients who dropped out of treatment (two or fewer therapy sessions) were slightly lower on the action scale, a finding consistent with the scale's intent.

Treatment group equivalence

Did randomization produce treatment groups that were equivalent on pretreatment characteristics? Table 5.2 shows the results of contrasting the four disulfiram-eligible groups on the primary measures of screening and diagnosis at intake, motivation for change, and drinking consumption and problems. Of 14 one-way ANOVAs, only two contrasts surpassed $p < 0.05$. The traditional group without disulfiram monitoring (Group 1) had somewhat lower MAST scores, a severity difference not corroborated by measures of alcohol dependence. Clients assigned to the CRA with the disulfiram-compliance condition (Group 3) reported, on average, more

Table 5.2. *Comparison of baseline drinking characteristics by assigned treatment condition: disulfiram-eligible clients (Groups 1–4)*

	Group 1 (n = 39)	Group 2 (n = 40)	Group 3 (n = 40)	Group 4 (n = 38)	F-test p
Screening and diagnosis					
Dependence (ADS)	15.3 (8.3)	16.8 (10.5)	15.9 (7.2)	17.6 (9.4)	0.70
Dependence (DSM)	6.67 (1.8)	7.2 (1.6)	6.9 (1.9)	6.9 (1.5)	0.58
MAST	22.0 (8.3)	26.3 (12.7)	27.3 (10.1)	28.7 (12.5)	0.05
Hamilton depression	6.6 (6.3)	8.5 (6.7)	6.3 (5.7)	8.1 (7.4)	0.36
Need for treatment (ASI)	3.3 (1.1)	3.4 (1.0)	3.5 (0.9)	3.3 (0.9)	0.77
Motivation for change					F-test p
Precontemplation	17.3 (5.4)	17.0 (7.2)	15.9 (5.5)	16.8 (6.4)	0.76
Contemplation	31.0 (5.6)	31.2 (5.5)	32.6 (4.3)	30.2 (3.5)	0.40
Determination	31.8 (6.8)	33.1 (6.5)	34.0 (5.5)	33.0 (5.4)	0.46
Action	31.8 (6.0)	33.5 (5.5)	32.8 (5.1)	33.3 (3.5)	0.47
Drinking and problems					F-test p
Years of problem	7.2 (5.5)	7.4 (6.3)	11.4 (6.6)	8.5 (7.2)	0.02
Alcohol problems	3.8 (3.1)	5.4 (4.3)	3.7 (2.9)	4.3 (3.5)	0.11
Maximum BAC	0.33 (0.19)	0.36 (0.19)	0.37 (0.18)	0.39 (0.19)	0.58
Standard drinks	712.2 (740.6)	734.9 (764.1)	706.5 (634.7)	785.5 (639.0)	0.96
Drinking days/week	4.3 (2.4)	4.3 (2.3)	3.8 (2.7)	4.1 (2.5)	0.79

Values are mean (SD).

years of problem drinking than did clients assigned to the other disulfiram-eligible conditions. This difference was not apparent on other measures of alcohol consumption and problem severity. Table 5.3 shows the parallel results contrasting the Traditional (Group 5) and CRA (Group 6) disulfiram-ineligible groups on the same measures. Here, none of the 14 one-way ANOVAs was significant. We conclude that the treatment groups were relatively well-balanced by randomization.

It is noteworthy, however, that on a wide variety of measures, disulfiram-ineligible clients (Groups 5 and 6) had problems of greater severity compared to disulfiram-eligible clients (Groups 1–4). For example, prior to randomization, disulfiram-ineligible clients were older ($p < 0.05$), drank on more days ($p < 0.002$), and reported significantly higher overall alcohol consumption ($p < 0.0002$) than disulfiram-eligible clients.

What about client satisfaction with treatment? We found no between-group differences in client global satisfaction with treatment (4-item scale) for Groups 1–4 [$F(1,125) = 2.31$, $p < 0.08$] or Groups 5 and 6 [$F(1,57) = 0.01, p < 0.91$]. Likewise, no between-group difference was found

Table 5.3. *Comparison of baseline drinking characteristics by assigned treatment condition: disulfiram-ineligible clients (Groups 5–6)*

	Group 5	Group 6	p
Screening and diagnosis			
Dependence (ADS)	15. 8 (9.2)	16.9 (9.0)	0.60
Dependence (DSM)	7.2 (1.5)	6.9 (1.9)	0.46
MAST	28.6 (1.3)	28.2 (9.7)	0.87
Hamilton depression	8.6 (5.6)	7.6 (6.0)	0.46
Need for treatment (ASI)	3.3 (1.2)	3.6 (0.7)	0.19
Readiness for change			
Precontemplation	16.5 (6.0)	15.5 (4.6)	0.42
Contemplation	32.3 (6.7)	31.6 (3.8)	0.40
Determination	33.3 (5.1)	34.8 (4.5)	0.15
Action	31.4 (5.5)	32.2 (5.6)	0.53
Drinking and problems			
Years of alcohol problems	7.6 (5.5)	9.6 (7.7)	0.20
Total alcohol problems	5.0 (3.3)	5.4 (3.5)	0.59
Maximum BAC	0.39 (0.19)	0.38 (0.18)	0.73
Total standard drinks/90 days	1206.3 (1091.5)	1047.4 (726.4)	0.44
Drinking days/week	5.1 (2.7)	5.4 (2.3)	0.59

ASI, Addiction Severity Index.

in ratings of therapists (5-item scale) for the two disulfiram-ineligible conditions [Groups 5 and 6, $F(1, 57) = 0.89$, $p < 0.5$]. Systematic group differences in therapist quality ratings, however, were found among the four disulfiram-eligible conditions [$F(3,120) = 4.98$, $p < 0.003$]. Here, clients assigned to Group 1, on average, rated their therapist significantly less favorably than did clients assigned to Groups 2 and 3. That is, the Traditional therapists were rated less favorably than the CRA therapists, even when the latter were delivering Traditional treatment (in Group 2).

Post hoc analyses indicated that global satisfaction with treatment and specific ratings of therapist qualities were powerful predictors of treatment outcome. Clients more satisfied with the treatment received and their therapist's abilities tended to drink significantly less often throughout follow-up (range of correlations, -0.19, $p < 0.01$ to -0.35, $p < 0.001$), reported drinking significantly lower total amounts of alcohol (range of correlations, -0.21, $p < 0.006$ to -0.41, $p < 0.001$), and, when they did drink, had significantly lower BAC estimates (range of correlations, -0.25, $p < 0.001$ to -0.35, $p < 0.001$).

Treatment compliance and fidelity

An important question is whether proportionally the same number of clients received an adequate *dose* of treatment to make post-treatment comparisons meaningful. It is also important to establish the intended distinctiveness of each treatment. Table 5.4 provides findings that address these two questions.

As shown, the same proportion of clients completed three or more sessions of therapy in the four disulfiram-eligible conditions [χ^2 (3) = 1.73, $p < 0.63$]. Likewise, no mean differences were found among the four groups in the total number of therapy sessions attended [$F(3,156) = 0.52, p < 0.67$]. This was not the case, however, in the two disulfiram-ineligible groups. Significantly fewer clients assigned to Traditional therapy completed three or more sessions, relative to disulfiram-ineligible clients assigned to CRA [χ^2 (1) = 12.06, $p < 0.001$]. These two groups demonstrated both the highest and the lowest therapy completion rates of the study. No difference was found in the mean number of therapy sessions attended by these two groups [$F(1,79) = 0.73, p < 0.40$], suggesting that the group difference was in the rate of early drop-outs (41% in traditional treatment versus 7% in CRA).

The taking and monitoring of disulfiram were important distinguishing aspects of the treatment groups (see Table 5.4). A significant difference in proportions was found among the four disulfiram-eligible groups in acceptance of disulfiram [χ^2 (3) = 36.99, $p < 0.001$], with a very high rate (90%) of acceptance in Group 2 (Traditional treatment with the CRA disulfiram-compliance procedure), and a low rate (18%) in Group 4 in which disulfiram was not prescribed as part of the treatment. Groups 1–4 also differed significantly in the proportion of clients with a disulfiram monitor. Only one client in Group 1 (Traditional treatment, without procedures to engage a monitor) reported having a significant other who helped ensure his taking disulfiram. The two groups with disulfiram-monitoring procedures (Groups 2 and 3) did not differ from each other in the rate of engaging a monitor [χ^2 (1) = 3.19, $p < 0.07$]. Thus the treatments did differ as intended in regard to acquiring disulfiram monitors.

This monitoring difference was also manifest in different rates of disulfiram compliance, measured as continuous rather than categorical variables. One-way ANOVAs indicated that the clients in the two monitoring conditions (combined) took disulfiram on significantly more days than did those in the two nonmonitoring groups combined [$F(1,109) = 11.05$,

Table 5.4. *Treatment attendance and disulfiram compliance*

	Assigned group					
	Disulfiram-eligible					Disulfiram-ineligible
	1	2	3	4	5	6
Treatment received						
% Complete[1]	76.9%	85.0%	87.5%	81.6%	58.8%	91.3%
Mean sessions	9.5 (7.6)	7.9 (5.3)	9.0 (6.5)	9.6 (7.0)	7.3 (7.2)	8.7 (7.1)
Mean cancels	2.3 (2.0)	3.5 (2.8)	3.4 (2.8)	4.0 (3.1)	2.7 (2.1)	3.8 (2.5)
Disulfiram compliance						
% Accepted[2]	51.3%	90.0%	56.4%	18.4%	–	–
% Monitored[3]	3.8%	48.7%	28.9%	18.8%[5]	–	–
% Compliant[4]	50.0%	80.6%	44.1%	44.4%	–	–
Mean refills	0.03 (0.17)	2.11 (2.05)	1.79 (2.77)	1.00 (1.31)	–	–
Mean % days	10.4 (14.6)	56.3 (60.5)	52.4 (84.4)	41.7 (43.6)	–	–

[1] Percentage of clients attending three or more therapy sessions.
[2] Percentage of clients accepting disulfiram prescription.
[3] Percentage of clients with a disulfiram monitor.
[4] Percentage of clients rated by therapists as disulfiram compliant.
[5] n too small for meaningful analysis.

$p < 0.001$], and refilled disulfiram prescriptions significantly more often than did the nonmonitoring groups [$F(1,109) = 20.05, p < 0.0001$]. The two Groups (2 and 3) with monitoring, however, did not differ from each other in terms of days of disulfiram use [$t(73) = -0.31, p < 0.76$].

In sum, with regard to treatment retention, proportionally the same number of clients assigned to the four disulfiram-eligible conditions completed three or more sessions. Conditions that were intended to initiate disulfiram monitoring did so, albeit not in all cases. In turn, clients receiving treatment that included monitoring took disulfiram on significantly more days and refilled more prescriptions than those who were not monitored. In the disulfiram-ineligible groups, differential early drop-out rates were found, but no difference was observed in the total number of therapy sessions attended by the two treatment groups.

Study follow-up rates

The validity of conclusions about treatment effectiveness depends in part on the extent to which enrolled clients are successfully interviewed during the follow-up phase of the study. It is also highly desirable for the attrition from follow-up across treatment groups to be similar. Table 5.5 shows the

Table 5.5. *Study follow-up rates: method of contact and reasons for no contact*

	Month of scheduled interview after recruitment							
	2	3	4	6	9	12	18	24
Interviewed (*n*)								
In person	75	69	76	66	33	53	68	122
Telephone	52	54	68	74	84	61	64	46
Home visit	0	0	0	0	0	3	7	18
Reconstruct	0	7	10	32	38	43	26	0
Not interviewed (*n*)								
Deceased	1	1	2	2	3	5	6	7
Incarcerated	3	6	7	4	6	10	7	4
Residential treatment	1	0	1	1	4	2	0	1
Refused	7	10	11	18	16	14	20	26
Lost	98	90	62	40	53	46	39	13
Monthly follow-up rate (%)								
Unadjusted	54	55	65	73	65	68	70	79
Adjusted[1]	55	57	68	75	69	73	74	83

[1] Denominator adjusted for deceased, incarcerated, and residential treatment clients.

number of clients interviewed at each of the eight follow-up points, and the method used to interview them. Also included in Table 5.5 are the reasons for and frequencies of no client contact. As shown, most client interviews were conducted in person or by telephone. Interviews identified as reconstructions are data that were reconstructed when a prior follow-up had been missed and the client was subsequently contacted and interviewed.

Chi-square tests were conducted to determine whether there was differential follow-up according to treatment condition. These were carried out at each of the eight follow-up intervals, and separately for Groups 1–4 and Groups 5–6. For the disulfiram-eligible clients, the eight 2 (interviewed versus not interviewed) by 4 (Groups 1–4) chi squares were all nonsignificant (smallest obtained p value $= 0.19$ at 2-month follow-up). For the disulfiram-ineligible clients, a differential follow-up rate (chi square at unprotected $p < 0.05$) was detected at the 6-month follow-up only, with proportionally fewer clients assigned to traditional therapy being inter-viewed, $p < 0.04$. Given that only one test of 16 yielded $p < 0.05$ without correction of α for multiple tests, we deemed this single finding to be, at most, a relatively minor threat to the integrity of the treatment compari-sons.

As described above, our follow-up rate for each of the early monthly interviews was low. As the difficulties with follow-up attrition became apparent and procedures were adjusted, the follow-up rate stabilized around 70%, finally reaching 83% (adjusted for deceased, incarcerated, and institutionalized clients) at the longest (24 months) follow-up point. To include a substantial proportion of clients in the statistical analyses of post-treatment functioning, we computed two time frames, proximal and distal follow-up points. The proximal follow-up period consisted of data collected at the 2-, 3-, and 4-month interviews. If clients were successfully interviewed at more than one of these months, their data were averaged by the number of interviews conducted. An analogous strategy was used for the 18- and 24-month follow-ups. This procedure yielded data at proximal follow-up for 82% of the total sample ($n = 194$) and for 84% of the total sample at the distal follow-up period.

Treatment effectiveness

The analyses reported above generally support the internal validity of this study, indicating that treatment comparisons of interest can be made with reasonable confidence. The *a priori* treatment contrasts were made at proximal and distal follow-up points using three primary dependent measures. The three outcome measures were total standard drinks con-sumed during the assessment period, number of drinking days per week, and estimated peak BAC for the assessment period. Four planned treat-ment contrasts were specified (see Chapter 4), each of which was tested at these two post-treatment periods. To reduce the need to protect against type I error, we elected to conduct four MANCOVAs at proximal follow-up, jointly using the three dependent measures pooled across months 1–6. At distal follow-up, the same four MANCOVAs were conducted, this time using data pooled across the 18- and 24-month follow-ups. Covariates in the analyses were baseline measures of the three primary dependent variables.

Prior to analyses the distributional characteristics of the three depend-ent measures were examined. This examination evaluated baseline, proximal, and distal distributions. Eleven outlier cases (SD > 3) were identified within Groups 1–4 across the six distributions (three baseline and three proximal) and were removed from analyses. In addition, two cases were removed from the analyses (Groups 1–4) because interview data had been collected either too early to be representative of proximal functioning (22 days after study recruitment) or too late to be considered representative of distal functioning (3 years post-treatment). Six other outlier cases were identified in Groups 1–4 using the three distal distributions. If a case was a statistical outlier in the proximal distributions but not in the distal or baseline distributions, the case was retained for the distal outcome analyses. Similar distributional analyses for clients assigned to Groups 5 and 6 yielded two outlier cases in the proximal distributions and one statistical outlier in the distal distributions.

Prospective statistical testing relied upon the intention-to-treat (ITT) sample: all clients, regardless of whether they received or did not receive the assigned therapy (three or more sessions), were included in the analyses if they provided the necessary post-treatment data. Parallel statistical tests including only the treated sample (clients with three or more sessions) were conducted and are also reported, but these analyses were *post hoc* and did not protect against an inflated type I error rate resulting from multiple contrasts. Prospective tests were protected against an inflated type I error rate by using a Bonferroni adjustment of alpha ($\alpha = 0.05/4 = 0.0125$) to account for conducting four MANCOVAs.

Outcomes for disulfiram-eligible clients

Table 5.6 provides the means (SD) for the three primary dependent measures for the four disulfiram-eligible groups at proximal and distal follow-up, in both the ITT and treated samples. The first prospective contrast involved combining the two CRA groups (3 and 4) and determining whether their pooled scores differed from the scores of clients assigned to traditional therapy without disulfiram compliance training (Group 1). This MANCOVA was significant [$F(3,81) = 9.98$, $p < 0.001$], indicating that, on average, clients receiving CRA differed in their drinking status at proximal follow-up relative to clients assigned to traditional therapy without disulfiram compliance. *Post hoc* testing indicated that the CRA clients drank on significantly fewer days than did clients in traditional treatment [$F(1,83) = 17.10$, $p < 0.001$], but that CRA and traditional therapy clients did not differ in their intensity of drinking, as measured by the peak BAC

Table 5.6. *Drinking outcomes for disulfiram-eligible clients (Groups 1–4)*

	Group 1	Group 2	Group 3	Group 4
Approach				
	Traditional	Traditional	CRA	CRA
Disulfiram?				
	No	Yes	Yes	No
Proximal follow-up (months 1–6)				
Intention-to-treat sample				
$n =$	30	32	29	29
Mean total drinks	69.2 (105.0)	25.0 (61.5)	42.9 (65.4)	61.4 (144.2)
Mean maximum BAC	0.14 (0.18)	0.12 (0.18)	0.19 (0.21)	0.22 (0.24)
Mean drink days/week	1.35 (1.94)	0.25 (0.59)	0.20 (0.43)	0.22 (0.65)
% Cases abstinent	41.9%	58.8%	34.4%	32.3%
Treated sample				
$n =$	25	31	26	27
Mean total drinks	48.9 (84.3)	25.8 (62.4)	41.0 (62.8)	40.9 (84.7)
Mean maximum BAC	0.12 (0.18)	0.12 (0.18)	0.18 (0.20)	0.22 (0.23)
Mean drink days/week	1.00 (1.55)	0.25 (0.60)	0.19 (0.42)	0.24 (0.67)
% Cases abstinent	46.2%	57.6%	35.7%	33.3%
Distal follow-up (months 16–24)				
Distal follow-up (months 16–24)				
Intention-to-treat sample				
$n =$	30	33	32	28
Mean total drinks	191.0 (262.0)	128.4 (152.2)	242.8 (291.7)	231.7 (260.7)
Mean maximum BAC	0.25 (0.21)	0.22 (0.22)	0.22 (0.19)	0.29 (0.24)
Mean drink days/week	1.75 (2.22)	1.21 (1.51)	2.06 (2.65)	1.66 (2.20)
% Cases abstinent	25.8%	25.7%	27.3%	27.6%
Treated sample				
$n =$	25	28	29	25
Mean total drinks	144.3 (234.6)	129.1 (151.8)	234.7 (281.4)	206.4 (231.1)
Mean maximum BAC	0.22 (0.19)	0.22 (0.21)	0.23 (0.19)	0.27 (0.23)
Mean drink days/week	1.36 (1.93)	1.32 (1.58)	1.98 (2.65)	1.64 (2.14)
% Cases abstinent	26.9%	23.3%	27.6%	28.0%

variable, or in the total number of drinks consumed during the proximal period. A secondary analysis was conducted to test this hypothesis by removing all abstinent cases and repeating treatment comparisons, this time using only data from clients who drank during proximal follow-up. The MANCOVA contrasting CRA groups with Group 1 again indicated that if clients did drink, those in traditional treatment drank significantly more often [$F(3, 47) = 12.06, p < 0.001$].

The second prospective contrast asked whether adding disulfiram monitoring to traditional treatment (Group 2) improved client outcome relative to traditional treatment without monitoring (Group 1). This MANCOVA narrowly missed statistical significance by the conservative adjusted alpha standard of $p < 0.0125$ [$F(3,55) = 3.72, p < 0.017$]. *Post hoc* study of the three dependent measures indicated that the traditional group receiving disulfiram monitoring tended to drink on fewer days ($p < 0.004$) and consumed somewhat fewer standard drinks during the entire proximal period ($p < 0.06$) compared with clients not receiving disulfiram monitoring. Adding disulfiram to traditional treatment appeared to suppress drinking, although it must also be remembered that different therapists treated these two groups.

The third prospective contrast involved the traditional group receiving compliance training (Group 2) and the CRA group receiving compliance training (Group 3). This MANCOVA was not significant [$F(3,54) = 1.59, p < 0.20$], and nor were any of the univariate tests of the three dependent measures (smallest obtained $p = 0.18$). Thus, in the context of the two earlier contrasts it appeared that adding CRA procedures to disulfiram training did not improve treatment outcome.

The fourth contrast examined CRA plus disulfiram-compliance training (Group 3) and CRA without disulfiram training (Group 4). Treatment outcome at proximal follow-up did not differ between these two groups [$F(3,51) = 0.12, p < 0.95$]. Thus, the outcomes of CRA treatment were not improved by the addition of disulfiram-compliance procedures.

The same four MANCOVAs were repeated, this time using only data for those clients attending three or more therapy sessions. Results were wholly consistent with the ITT analyses. In particular, traditional therapy without compliance training (Group 1) fared significantly more poorly than the combined CRA treatments (3 and 4) [$F(3,71) = 7.43, p < 0.001$] at proximal follow-up. Likewise, the contrast between compliance training with traditional therapy (Group 2) and traditional therapy without training (Group 1) did not reach protected significance either [$F(3,49) = 2.79$,

$p < 0.05$]. As before, the two groups appeared to differ in terms of the frequency of drinking measure [$F(1,51) = 5.94$, $p < 0.018$]. Finally, neither contrast three nor contrast four obtained statistical significance.

When these prospective MANCOVAs were repeated with distal follow-up data, none of the contrasts attained even unprotected statistical significance (all p values >0.05). Prospective testing indicated that mean differences among the four groups reflected chance variation and were unrelated to treatment assignment. Likewise, none of the four MANCOVAs based upon treated cases (three or more therapy sessions) attained protected or unprotected statistical significance, nor did any of the univariate tests.

A question of interest that was not addressed by the planned contrasts is whether the groups differed from one another in the rate of *complete* abstinence during follow-up. Using all available data, clients were classified to either an abstinent group or a drinking group during proximal and distal follow-up months. Any evidence indicating even a single drink during the follow-up period led to their assignment to the drinking category. Cases that had been identified as extreme outliers and eliminated from prior prospective analyses were included in this category analyses. Rates of complete abstinence for Groups 1–4 are included in Table 5.6. Chi-square tests were used to replicate the four planned contrasts with treatment group as one dimension (1 degree of freedom, df) and drinking status as the second dimension (1 df). None of these was significant at $p < 0.0125$ (protected for four tests), and only one surpassed $p < 0.05$: at proximal follow-up only, clients assigned to traditional treatment with disulfiram-compliance training (Group 2) reported a higher rate of abstinence than did clients receiving CRA and compliance training (Group 3).

Outcomes for disulfiram-ineligible clients

How did the CRA and traditional treatments compare at follow-up for disulfiram-*ineligible* clients? Table 5.7 reports the mean (SD) of the two groups at proximal and distal follow-ups. As before, the difference in the number of clients reported between the ITT and treated analyses indicates the proportion of clients not receiving an adequate dose of treatment. Earlier analyses had indicated the presence of a differential rate of treatment exposure (three or more sessions) between these two groups, with greater drop-out in traditional treatment. This finding is clearly illustrated in Table 5.7. At proximal follow-up, neither ITT nor the treated sample analyses

Table 5.7. *Drinking outcomes for disulfiram-ineligible clients (Groups 5–6)*

	Group 5 Traditional	Group 6 CRA
	Proximal follow-up (months 1–6)	
Intention-to-treat sample		
$n =$	24	36
Mean total standard drinks	83.90 (117.66)	103.31 (153.19)
Mean maximum BAC	0.19 (0.20)	0.26 (0.21)
Mean drinking days per week	1.69 (2.37)	1.68 (2.40)
Percent cases abstinent	24.0%	22.2%
Treated sample		
$n =$	18	32
Mean total standard drinks	72.71 (112.61)	99.10 (153.28)
Mean maximum BAC	0.19 (0.20)	0.24 (0.20)
Mean drinking days per week	1.20 (1.89)	1.53 (2.27)
Percent cases abstinent	33.3%	21.1%
	Distal follow-up (months 16–24)	
Intention-to-treat sample		
$n =$	29	35
Mean total standard drinks	254.27 (339.49)	266.76 (357.40)
Mean maximum BAC	0.26 (0.23)	0.28 (0.21)
Mean drinking days per week	1.72 (2.39)	2.00 (2.30)
Percent cases abstinent	31.0%	22.2%
Treated sample		
$n =$	17	31
Mean total standard drinks	245.88 (365.24)	242.45 (292.15)
Mean maximum BAC	0.23 (0.24)	0.27 (0.22)
Mean drinking days per week	1.79 (2.64)	1.98 (2.21)
Percent cases abstinent	35.3%	25.0%

were significant using the MANCOVA approach described earlier. Likewise, no therapy group difference was found at distal follow-up with either the ITT or the treated groups. Exploratory analyses further indicated that none of the *post hoc* univariate tests using the three dependent measures distinguished between the two disulfiram-ineligible groups.

Similarly, complete abstinence rates (see Table 5.7) did not differ between Groups 5 and 6 [χ^2 (1) = 0.03, $p < 0.87$]. An obvious difference is the lower rate of abstinence during proximal follow-up among disulfiram-ineligible clients, regardless of treatment condition, relative to those shown in Table 5.6. Collapsing across treatments, this chi square indicated that proportionally more disulfiram-eligible clients (41.2%) were completely abstinent during proximal follow-up than disulfiram-ineligible clients (23.0%) [χ^2 (1) = 6.92, $p < 0.009$].

Post hoc *power analyses*

A *post hoc* power analysis was conducted to determine the relative likelihood of the planned contrasts rejecting the null hypothesis. On average, each study cell contained 30 clients, and conservatively we estimated obtaining a moderate effect size of 0.25. Assuming a type I error rate of 0.05, a single *df* contrast using four cells had a statistical power of 0.78, whereas a contrast based upon three cells ($n = 90$) had 0.65 power. In a three-cell contrast a slightly larger effect size of 0.30 (still far below the effect sizes reported in studies from the Azrin group) yielded a statistical power in excess of 0.80. Finally, in a two-cell contrast an effect size of 0.35 was required to obtain a statistical power of 0.76.

How did the effect sizes observed in the present study compare with the magnitude of changes reported by Azrin's group? Exact calculation of an effect size proved difficult for the Azrin et al. (1976) study because of sketchy statistical reporting. An effect size of 1.9 can be conservatively estimated given the probability values of the reported independent *t*-tests ($df = 17$). This estimate assumes a two-tailed test, and adequate statistical power ($\beta = 0.76$). By any standards, this difference in drinking reduction is dramatic and would strongly recommend the CRA approach over traditional therapy. Effects were considerably smaller in our study, but nonetheless support CRA as being more effective than traditional therapy. Specifically, two of the four planned contrasts compared CRA-related procedures with traditional therapy. Effect sizes favoring the CRA procedures were 0.94 (cell one versus cell two) and 0.77 (cell one versus cells three and four) for reductions in drinks per drinking occasion at proximal follow-up. These effects were derived using Hedges' and Olkin's (1985) formula for calculating unbiased effect estimates. Could sampling error alone explain differences between Azrin's reported effect size and our own? Computation of a grand mean effect size with 95% confidence intervals (mean = 1.11, 95% confidence interval = 0.60–1.62) indicated that the effect sizes were not homogenous, and specifically that the effect size reported by Azrin ($d = 1.9$) was significantly larger than the effects reported here (Hedges & Olkin, 1985). Thus, while the effects in this study were significantly smaller than those reported by Azrin et al. (1976), treatment effects in this study were nevertheless large in magnitude, and consistent in direction with Azrin's evaluations of CRA.

Did a lack of statistical power limit our ability to detect the contributions made by components of CRA? Estimated effect sizes for contrasting disulfiram monitoring plus traditional treatment with disulfiram monitoring plus CRA yielded an effect size of 0.08 on the drinks per drinking day measure at proximal follow-up, and an effect size of 0.004 was obtained between CRA with and without disulfiram monitoring for the same measure at proximal follow-up. There was no evidence of a narrow miss here; the estimated effects were quite small, and unlikely to be of clinical significance.

Overall reductions in drinking

At the longer follow-up points of 18 and 24 months, no differences remained among treatment groups. As is evident from a comparison of Tables 5.6 and 5.7, some of this is due to an increase in the overall quantity and frequency of drinking from proximal to distal months. Nevertheless, substantial changes in drinking remained. Collapsing across all six treatment groups at distal follow-up, relative to baseline, there was a 75% reduction in both the frequency (effect size = −1.18) and the quantity of drinking (effect size = −0.97). These reductions were sufficiently large that, despite sizeable variances, there was no overlap of the confidence intervals for baseline and follow-up means.

Post hoc *exploratory analyses*

Further analyses were conducted to address three questions: (1) how reliable were client self-reports? (2) did therapists differ in their effectiveness? (3) did client attributes predict differential responsiveness to treatments?

1. *Reliability of self-reports*

Collateral interviews were conducted to assess the veracity of self-reported use of alcohol. To this end, 153 collaterals were interviewed at intake. While collateral interviews were conducted at all points parallel to client follow-up interviews, statistical comparisons of client and collateral reports of client drinking were made at the 4-month (81 collateral–client pairs) and 24-month (55 collateral–client pairs) follow-ups. These time points were selected because of their centrality to planned primary outcome analyses. Significant and positive correlations were obtained for all three measures of drinking at all three comparison points. At intake, 4, and 24 months, collateral–client correlations were positive and significant for the number of drinking days per week ($r = 0.34$, 0.36, and 0.30), for number of standard drinks consumed ($r = 0.50$, 0.48, and 0.86), and for average drinks per week ($r = 0.37$, 0.53, and 0.43), respectively. Yet another method to assess the client report is to dichotomize self-reported alcohol use (drinking versus abstinent) and to compare this transformed variable with the collateral report of client abstinence and/or drinking. Examined at proximal follow-up (months 2–4), we found that 40% of the collateral–client pairs agreed that the client was not drinking and 31% of the pairs were in agreement that the client had been drinking (71% exact agreement). Another 10% of clients reported drinking while their collateral reported abstinence. Finally, 18% of collaterals reported that the client had some alcohol while the client reported no alcohol use. (The latter cases were counted as nonabstinent in computation of group rates of complete abstinence.)

2. Therapist effects

Analyses were conducted to determine whether therapists differed in their effectiveness as measured by client drinking outcomes during follow-up. For stable estimates of therapist effects we included in analyses only therapists who had treated a minimum of ten clients (cf. Project MATCH Research Group, 1998). Four therapists met this criterion, three of whom were CRA therapists. We elected to remove the one traditional therapist from analyses because this would have confounded tests of therapist effectiveness with treatment group assignment. MANCOVAs were conducted with the therapist as a between-subject factor (three levels) and the baseline value of the dependent measure as a covariate. Dependent measures included both process and drinking measures. No difference was obtained in the number of treatment sessions attended [$F(2,151) = 1.97$, $p < 0.14$], although one therapist did have significantly fewer canceled therapy appointments [$F(2,150) = 5.97$, $p < 0.003$]. The number of client cancellations, however, was not significantly related to treatment outcome.

No differences were found among the three CRA therapists in terms of client drinking outcomes at proximal or distal follow-up.

3. Matching effects

Finally, we analyzed for client–treatment matching effects, seeking to identify those pretreatment client attributes that predicted a differential responsiveness to treatments. Exploratory analyses were conducted for gender, marital status, readiness for change, and severity of drinking problem. No support was found for a differential treatment response based upon these client characteristics, although it must be noted that the statistical power for testing these interaction effects was poor.

Discussion

What can be concluded from the findings of this clinical trial? First, *the treatments tested appeared to be equally acceptable to clients.* On average, clients completed about nine sessions (75%) of all treatments, with no differences in retention based on traditional versus CRA or emphasis on disulfiram. The anomaly here was a high rate of early drop-out (41%) from traditional treatment among the more severe disulfiram-ineligible clients, as compared with a low drop-out rate (9%) for the same group given CRA. This difference in retention was not mirrored, however, in better outcomes for the CRA group.

Second, among disulfiram-eligible clients, those who received CRA treatment drank on significantly fewer days during their proximal follow-up (months 1–6), as compared with clients given traditional treatment. The difference was large ($p < 0.001$), with 3% drinking days in CRA groups versus 19% drinking days in traditional treatment. *CRA thus was found to be more successful in suppressing the frequency of drinking, as compared with traditional treatment without disulfiram monitoring, during the first 6 months after intake.*

Third, among disulfiram-eligible clients in months 1–6, about the same high degree of benefit (4% drinking days) was obtained when traditional treatment was combined with the disulfiram-compliance procedures from CRA. That is, outcomes in traditional treatment were as good as those with the full CRA treatment when the therapist engaged a significant other to help the client monitor and adhere to disulfiram medication. In this group, 90% accepted disulfiram, with 81% compliance (by therapist report), and self-report indicated that disulfiram was taken on the greatest number of days compared to the other groups, even though a significant-other monitor was successfully engaged in only half of the cases. *In the presence of disulfiram monitoring, CRA and traditional treatment did not differ in efficacy.*

Fourth, within CRA-treated groups of clients eligible to take disulfiram, we found similar outcomes with and without disulfiram. This comparison was marred by the fact that only 56% of clients in the CRA plus disulfiram (Group 3) accepted disulfiram, and only 29% had a significant other trained as a monitor. This is particularly puzzling in that the same CRA therapists were quite successful with disulfiram compliance in Group 2, suggesting that the taking of disulfiram may be more consonant (at least in the clients' minds) with a disease model than with a behavioral approach. Traditional and CRA groups also had similar outcomes among the disulfiram-ineligible clients. *The addition of disulfiram-monitoring procedures did not significantly increase the efficacy of CRA.*

Fifth, *adding disulfiram-compliance procedures significantly improved proximal outcomes in traditional treatment.* It must be noted here that in order to avoid contamination of Group 1, different therapists conducted traditional treatment without (Group 1) and with disulfiram-compliance procedures (Group 2), and that high abstinence rates were characteristic of clients in all three groups treated by the CRA therapists, whether they were delivering traditional (with disulfiram, Group 2) or CRA treatment (Groups 3 and 4). Thus therapists were confounded with the presence versus absence of disulfiram monitoring in traditional treatment Groups 1 and 2. If Group 2 therapists were more effective than Group 1 therapists, this could account for the observed difference, although no outcome difference was observed between the same two groups of therapists delivering treatment to Groups 5 and 6.

Sixth, when perfect continuous abstinence in months 1–6 was examined, *traditional treatment* (Group 2) *relative to CRA* (Group 3) *in the presence of disulfiram yielded a somewhat higher rate of total abstention* (59% versus 34% continuously abstinent), with both treatments administered by the same therapists. This difference failed to reach statistical significance, however, with protection against type I error in multiple tests. When traditionally treated clients did drink, they drank significantly more often than CRA-treated clients – a finding consistent with the abstinence viol-ation effect associated with a disease model of alcoholism.

Finally, a high rate of recurrence of drinking was observed in all groups by distal follow-up. Continuous abstinence during these months declined to about 30%. *No between-group differences on outcome measures endured at 2 years.*

Did we replicate Azrin's findings? In many respects, we did. CRA was associated with a nearly complete suppression of drinking during months 1–6, the period of follow-up reported in Azrin's outpatient study. Adding disulfiram-compliance alone to traditional treatment yielded benefits comparable to those for the full CRA package – a finding that was restricted to married clients in Azrin's study. Our CRA groups also drank substantially less frequently than traditionally treated clients, although the absolute magnitude of difference was not as large as that reported by Azrin et al. (1982).

A question unanswered by Azrin's studies is whether disulfiram is *necessary* for the efficacy of CRA for clients who can take this medication. Our data indicate that it is not. Indeed, the original CRA study (Hunt & Azrin, 1973) reported excellent outcomes without the use of disulfiram. It appears, therefore, that when effective behavioral treatment is offered, the use of disulfiram is not essential.

We also have some findings that are discrepant with results reported by Azrin and his colleagues. The CRA-trained therapists in this study showed similarly favorable outcomes whether delivering CRA or traditional treatment (with disulfiram monitoring). In the Azrin et al. study (1982), the same behaviorally trained therapists delivered both CRA and traditional treatments, but with CRA treatment leading to a substantially better outcome. Among the more severely impaired clients in the disulfiram-ineligible arm of our study, we found no difference between CRA and traditional treatment, a finding at variance with the Azrin studies reviewed in Chapter 2.

When we used the traditional outcome standard of *continuous* abstinence, we found a somewhat higher percentage of abstinent clients in Group 2 (traditional treatment with disulfiram compliance) than in Group 3 (CRA with disulfiram compliance) during proximal follow-up, even though both were treated by the same therapists. This finding directly parallels the report from Project MATCH (1997) that, despite a lack of difference on other outcome metrics, a significantly higher proportion of outpatients abstained continuously when given a 12-step facilitation treatment, compared to those offered cognitive-behavioral treatment. One obvious explanation is that total abstinence (and relatedly, the use of disulfiram) is consistent with the central tenets of the disease-model rationale emphasized in our traditional treatment. Abstinence was also encouraged in the groups receiving CRA, but it may be that a behavioral approach with its emphasis on self-management is less likely to inspire complete abstinence. In the language of self-efficacy, a traditional approach seeks to enhance self-efficacy for abstinence, while suppressing self-efficacy for moderation. Cognitive-behavioral approaches tend to emphasize self-control more generally, enhancing efficacy for the management of one's own behavior. It would be expected, then, that a traditional treatment approach might be associated with a higher rate of perfect abstinence, but poorer self-management of drinking. A behavioral approach, in contrast, might not produce such a high rate of continuous abstinence, but when drinking occurs it may be more regulated. In our study, a significant difference was observed in the frequency of drinking days, with CRA-treated clients drinking less often than traditionally treated clients.

This study proved to be no simple horse race. Our findings varied with the severity of the sample treated (disulfiram eligible versus ineligible). CRA had better results than traditional treatment when outcome was measured in one way (frequency of drinking), but not on other measures of outcome (e.g., continuous abstinence). The addition of disulfiram compliance appears to have enhanced the efficacy of traditional treatment, but not that of CRA. Traditional and CRA treatments had similar outcomes when combined with disulfiram monitoring. Although all observed significant differences favored CRA over traditional treatment, there are indications in our findings that both disulfiram and a traditional approach can be useful. Indeed, by 2-year follow-up, no significant outcome differences endured.

We also, as in Project MATCH (1997), found no indication of strong client–treatment matches. That is, our data offer clinicians no clear guidelines for which kinds of clients should be assigned to CRA, to traditional treatment, or to disulfiram therapy. We are left with a familiar picture. Clinicians have at their disposal a menu of potentially effective treatment methods with which to help clients who have alcohol problems. We have no great wisdom for selecting the treatment approach that the clients should follow. The good news is that if one particular approach is unacceptable or ineffective for a client, there are alternatives available.

Pitfalls

The report of these findings has taken far longer than we anticipated. The last follow-up data were collected in 1991, and our progress since then has been a process of learning better ways to analyze (and conduct) treatment outcome research. Our current clinical trials reflect the greater methodological and practical experience compared to when we conducted this trial. We conclude this chapter, therefore, with a confessional litany of some errors we made along the way, in the hope of saving colleagues from similar pitfalls.

Error no. 1. Wait until the end of the study to enter the data

We gave priority in this study to recruiting clients, collecting data, and keeping the project running within protocol. Hard copy client data forms were stored in research files with the plan of entering them in batch form after data collection had concluded. This proved problematic in several respects. As frequently happens, recruitment and data collection took longer than expected. This pressed data entry even closer to the end of the funding period. By the time data were entered, most of the staff who had collected them had graduated, moved away to internship and employment, or moved on to other projects. This made it difficult to clarify illegible, discrepant, ambiguous, or missing information. Data entry also took longer than expected, and had to be completed by unfunded research assistants working for course credit. As indicated below, we ultimately had to re-enter the entire data set.

Error no. 2. Enter data once

We initially relied on the single entry of records by undergraduate student research assistants, with visual spot checking against case records. When our statistician (J.S.T.) began to analyze the data set, it became clear that there were serious errors. Out-of-range values appeared. Treatment conditions had been miscoded in some cases. There were duplicate records of the same case. True zero values had been recorded as missing data, and *vice versa*. We had no choice but to start again, bearing the cost of independent double-entry from overhead funds, and fitting it in between other projects. It set us back by more than a year. Now we routinely use independent double-entry with electronic comparison of records, entering data within 2 weeks of collection so that uncertain points can be clarified, missing data may be obtained, and problems with instruments and interviews can be quickly detected.

Error no. 3. Change staff in midstream

In the course of the trial we had three different project coordinators and a large number of graduate and undergraduate research assistants. This required constant retraining of new staff. Because data were not entered as the trial progressed, we were slow to catch poor interview completion rates for specific research assistants, resulting in lower than optimal rates of retention in follow-up. The third project coordinator (K.A.G.) detected the problem, and made heroic (and successful) efforts to improve the interview rates at the more distal follow-up points (to 24 months). We now use computer-based project tracking systems that generate monthly reports of the status of data collection and entry completion.

Error no. 4. Interview frequently

Our initial plan was to have clients return monthly for detailed interviews about their drinking. A good plan on paper, it proved quite challenging in practice – a difficulty encountered by other investigators as well (e.g., Sobell & Sobell, 1984). Clients simply balked at being interviewed this often. Consequently they proved difficult to schedule, with frequent cancellations and no-shows, and before one month's interview could be completed the next came due. This was exacerbated by an unanticipated problem with incentives. We had proposed to give clients a lottery draw ticket for immediate cash prizes each time they returned for follow-up, a cost-effective procedure we had previously used with success. What we did not realize is that this method works well – *once*. One empty envelope seemed to quickly extinguish the novel attraction (although the few winners did return faithfully for their next interview). We quickly developed a procedure of keeping each assessment window open until the day before the next follow-up came due, and of reconstructing data from missed follow-up points, a procedure that proved reasonably reliable (Grant et al., 1997). This created a few outlier dates, however, that had to be excluded from the analyses (as indicated above). We now retain experienced research staff across trials to perform the highly skilled functions of case tracking and structured interviewing.

Error no. 5. Assume therapists will follow procedures

Supervision in this trial relied on therapists' self-reports of what they did behind closed doors. We thought this reasonable, given that our traditional therapists were well set in their ways and committed to the disease-model and 12-step methods they were to deliver, while our CRA therapists were specifically trained and regularly supervised for purposes of the trial. We now know, however, that what therapists say they do may bear little resemblance to what is actually done, even when sessions are recorded. Subsequent clinical trials in which we audiotaped or videotaped all therapy sessions have taught us the amount of training and supervision that is required to maintain the integrity of treatment protocols. It is also the case that counselors most need help with the very things that they did not see and cannot report to their supervisor. While the ability to discriminate between treatments in this trial was supported by the protocol compliance data we did collect, and after the fact by observed differences in outcome, it would have been better to have more direct therapist adherence measures. Thus we now routinely record sessions for supervision and quality assurance purposes.

Error no. 6. Move on to other projects before the data have been analyzed

Despite the best of intentions, it can be vexing to come back to a data set a year or two after a study has been completed. First of all, investigators are probably involved in new projects that demand their time and attention. It becomes first difficult and then aversive to reconstruct exactly what was done, how the data set was organized, and what conventions were used in coding. New errors are found. Those who remember details may have moved away. Unless a faithful officer of the funding agency keeps asking for the report (as surely happened in this case: thank you to Drs. Richard Fuller and John Allen), it is easy to let sleeping data lie. We now include sufficient time and effort for data analysis in our project plans and funding applications.

From conducting this study we learned much that has improved our subsequent clinical trials. Psychotherapy outcome research is inherently complex, and we look forward to continued learning from future trials and errors.

6

CRA with the Homeless

JANE ELLEN SMITH AND HAROLD D. DELANEY

Homelessness in the United States

Although the homelessness problem in the United States has been apparent for many years, both the magnitude of the problem and its visibility have grown. Furthermore, the individuals who comprise the homeless population have changed dramatically. The "new" homeless are younger, better educated individuals who are commonly from minority ethnic groups. Additionally, today's homeless are more apt to have substance-abuse problems, mental illness, or both (Fischer, 1989; Fischer & Breakey, 1991; Rossi, 1990). Finally, there has also been a substantial increase in the number of homeless women and families, with this subgroup now constituting 25–30% of the total homeless population (Rossi, 1990; Welte & Barnes, 1992).

Given the highly heterogeneous nature of the homeless population and the many needs identified, the task of determining where to focus in order to effectively bring about change has been difficult for clinicians and researchers alike. Nevertheless, one consistent finding has emerged: alcoholism is the most widespread health problem of the homeless (Fischer, 1989; Institute of Medicine, 1988; Lubran, 1989). Probably the two best estimates of alcohol-use disorders within this population are 30–40% (McCarty et al., 1991) or even higher at 45–57% [National Institute on Alcohol Abuse and Alcoholism (NIAAA), 1991]. Furthermore, alcohol-dependent homeless individuals have more extreme problems than the rest of the homeless population in such areas as criminal arrests (Fischer, 1988; Gelberg, Linn & Leake, 1988), poor physical health (Wright & Weber, 1987), victimization (Geissler et al., 1995; NIAAA, 1992a), chronic unemployment (Koegel & Burnam, 1987), illegal drug use, and comorbid mental illness (NIAAA, 1991; Wright, 1989).

Treatment outcome research

Controlled trials specifically designed to test the efficacy of treatments for homeless individuals with alcohol problems were virtually nonexistent 10 years ago. A few studies focused on dually diagnosed individuals primarily (Drake & Wallach, 1989), or addressed the population's needs other than substance-abuse treatment (Caton et al., 1993). But a shift occurred in 1987 when the Stewart B. McKinney Homeless Assistance Act was introduced. This provided the funding for two rounds of demonstration projects through the NIAAA and the National Institute on Drug Abuse (NIDA). Ten of the projects provided data on individuals with alcohol as their primary drug. In brief, although alcohol use decreased more for treatment participants than for the comparison group, the differences were rarely significant.

With one exception, these demonstration projects utilized a case management program. The "exception", the Los Angeles program, was one of the few that showed significant between-group differences in substance abuse (Grella, 1993). However, the difference was found only when the records of those who actually attended the follow-up were examined, and not when the intention-to-treat sample was investigated. The experimental treatment condition consisted of both rural and urban residential recovery, and contained a combination of skills training and 12-step meetings. The comparison group received only the first residential phase. The somewhat promising results should be viewed with caution, however, because the follow-up rate was only 50%, assignment to condition was not entirely random, and treatment integrity could not be guaranteed.

Significant between-group differences were detected for only two of the nine case management projects. The Boston study (McCarty et al., 1990) found significant group differences in substance use, employment, and housing that favored the case management condition over customary aftercare. However, this only occurred when examining the "total sample", which assumed that individuals lost to follow-up did not improve. Given that the follow-up rate for the comparison group was only 59%, this assumption applied to many participants. Methodological limitations included contamination of the customary care condition with case management services, inclusion of only those individuals who had completed a 3-week stabilization program first, and the fact that case managers conducted their own follow-up interviews (NIAAA, 1992*b*). The second project that demonstrated significant group differences favoring case management over normal aftercare was conducted in Chicago (Sosin, Bruni & Reidy, 1995; Sosin & Yamaguchi, 1995). Interestingly, the case management condition included a cognitive-behavioral relapse component, and many of the basic necessities offered by the program (e.g., food vouchers, medical care) were contingent upon participants attending sessions. The study was limited by group assignment that only approached randomization, a requirement for participants to complete a 3- to 4-week stabilization period first, and a higher initial rejection rate for the one case management condition that did not include housing.

The results of the remaining demonstration projects are somewhat difficult to interpret, because although pre- to post-treatment improvements generally were found within conditions, there were no significant differences when case management was contrasted with the control group. This occurred when either "proactive" (Bonham et al., 1990) or intensive case management (Willenbring et al., 1990) was compared with standard levels of case management, when case management was contrasted with peer-supervised housing programs (Lapham, Hall & Skipper, 1995), or when intensive case management services were added to a standard substance-abuse program (Braucht et al., 1995). Perhaps contributing to this lack of differences were the many methodological limitations, including group assignment that was not entirely random, differential attrition rates across conditions, low follow-up rates, treatment contamination, baseline nonequivalence on demographic variables, and high drop-out rates. A recent study also utilized case management services with a homeless population, but this time the control group received no formal intervention (Toro et al., 1997). Significant between-group differences in support of the case management condition were only detected for quality of housing, level of psychopathology, and number of stressful events. Little improvement was found within the substance-abuse and employment areas. In summary, variations of case management services appear to be the standard approach for treating homeless individuals with alcohol problems. Unfortunately, the results from the studies that tested the efficacy of case management services were not compelling, and even the somewhat promising findings tended to deteriorate over time (Stahler, 1995).

Testing CRA with the homeless

In considering other suitable options for a substance-abuse treatment program for the homeless, one solid choice was the empirically based behavioral intervention called the Community Reinforcement Approach (CRA). CRA offers a comprehensive approach to substance-abuse treatment that addresses many of the needs of homeless men and women. Furthermore, its greatest relative treatment gains are obtained with its least socially stable clients (Azrin et al., 1982). With these factors in mind, we set out to compare two programs for alcohol-dependent homeless individuals: CRA and the standard treatment offered at a large day shelter (Smith, Meyers & Delaney, 1998). The traditional CRA program was modified to better suit the needs of the homeless population. These changes included: (1) adopting a group treatment format; (2) adding goal-setting and independent living skills groups; (3) adding a weekly community meeting as an opportunity for concerns to be voiced and for the Social Club activity to be decided; (4) offering a sizeable number of groups each week, thereby allowing for "misses" without jeopardizing treatment effectiveness; (5) using small incentives for attendance; and (6) allowing interested individuals to participate even if they were unwilling or unable to take disulfiram. Additionally, we housed individuals in both conditions throughout the program, since this seemed necessary in order to enable them to begin working on substance-abuse and employment problems.

Hypotheses

Our main hypothesis was that members of the CRA group would perform significantly better than control participants in terms of decreased alcohol consumption and increased employment and housing stability. A second interest was in determining whether the disulfiram component of the CRA program substantially enhances the efficacy of CRA treatment. It was expected to be an important supplement for this heavy drinking population, given that its daily administration by a monitor appears helpful in the early stages of treatment for impulsive drinkers with numerous treatment failures (Azrin et al., 1982). And so we hypothesized that CRA participants who received disulfiram as part of their treatment would reduce their drinking significantly more than CRA participants who did not receive it. However, since we anticipated that a fair number of potential participants would be opposed to taking disulfiram, or would have medical contraindications for its use, we instituted a five-condition design which allowed for a track assignment based on these considerations. This design allowed us to test whether an initial willingness to take disulfiram represented enhanced motivation, and whether medical ineligibility implied a serious, chronic drinking history that compromised treatment outcome. The prediction was that those assigned to the track for participants able and willing to take disulfiram would have an advantage over corresponding group members who were unwilling or unable.

The method

Participants

Chronic homeless adults participated in the project. We recruited them primarily at the largest day shelter program for the homeless in Albuquerque, New Mexico. Referrals also were accepted from the overnight shelters in town, from the state's inpatient detoxification facility, from an outpatient substance-abuse treatment program for indigents, and from the local Health Care for the Homeless program. Participants were diagnosable with alcohol dependence according to the *Diagnostic and statistical manual of mental disorders* (3rd edn., revised; DSM-III-R; American Psychiatric Association, 1987) at some point during the 6 months prior to intake. The Structured Clinical Interview for the DSM-III-R (SCID; Spitzer et al., 1988) was administered by an advanced graduate student in clinical psychology in order to establish the diagnosis. Potential participants were excluded for being: diagnosable with a primary drug problem other than alcohol ($n = 9$), involved full-time in a different substance-abuse program ($n = 5$), unable to supply the names of two collateral contacts ($n = 4$), unwilling to forgo starting a day job for 3 weeks in order to attend the treatment groups ($n = 4$), opposed to living in the grant-sponsored accommodations ($n = 4$), intoxicated for three contiguous assessment appointments ($n = 3$), actively psychotic ($n = 3$), not diagnosable with an alcohol problem ($n = 3$), or not homeless ($n = 1$).

A total of 213 potential participants inquired about the program. In addition to the 36 individuals noted above who were excluded, 71 were not enrolled because they failed to complete the assessment process. In two of these cases the individuals were hospitalized during the intake, and in 16 others the potential participants changed their minds after reading through the consent form. The reasons for the remaining 51 individuals failing to complete the assessment at various stages were unknown. Finally, and although initially considered eligible and included, data from two individuals were later eliminated when it became apparent that they had withheld information at intake that would have excluded them from the start. Thus, the final sample of legitimate participants who began treatment was 106. The "treated" sample consisted of 101 individuals, since five terminated the program prematurely.

In terms of the demographics for the 106 participants, there were 91 men (86%) and 15 women (14%). On average these individuals were 38 years old, with a range of 18–69 years. The average educational profile was that of a high school graduate. The ethnic breakdown was as follows: 64% White, 19% Hispanic, 13% Native American, and 4% African American. As far as marital status, a total of 97% were single. Among these, 49% were divorced or separated, 46% were never married, and 2% were widowed. Participants were largely unemployed at intake (91%), with the remainder reporting either a part-time (7%) or a full-time (2%) job.

Measures

Alcohol diagnosis and severity level

In addition to satisfying the DSM-III-R criteria for alcohol dependence sometime during the previous 6 months, participants were required to meet the recommended criteria for current dependence on at least one of three measures. These included: the Addiction Severity Index (ASI; McLellan et al., 1980), the Alcohol Use Inventory (AUI; Horn, Wanberg & Foster, 1987), and elevated gamma glutamyl transpeptidase (GGTP) liver enzymes.

Pretreatment characteristics

The primary instrument utilized to collect quantity and frequency information for substance use was the structured interview called the Brief Drinker Profile (BDP; Miller & Marlatt, 1987). The employment and legal status sections of the ASI (McLellan et al., 1980) were also administered. This instrument had been used successfully with other homeless populations (Argeriou et al., 1994; Drake, McHugo & Biesanz, 1995). A blood chemistry profile was also examined. In addition to the GGTP already mentioned, serum aspartate aminotransferase (AST, formerly known as glutamic oxalacetic transaminase, SGOT) and serum alanine aminotransferase (ALT, formerly known as glutamic pyruvic transaminase, SGPT) were used as dependent variables. Several other assessment instruments relevant to comorbidity issues were administered as part of this study but will not be reported here since the results have not yet been published.

Follow-up assessments

Follow-up interviews were conducted at 2, 4, 6, 9, and 12 months after the intake by research assistants who were advanced graduate students in clinical psychology. The research assistants discussed neither individual cases nor group assignment with the therapists, and consequently were uninformed regarding condition. Occasional exceptions to this occurred when a participant inadvertently divulged his or her treatment condition. The main instrument was the Follow-up Drinker Profile (FDP; Miller & Marlatt, 1984), which was the follow-up companion to the BDP. At the time of the 6- and 12-month follow-ups the ASI and the blood chemistry profiles were repeated as well. Participants were given $20 for each completed follow-up.

Treatment

Group assignment

The design of the study included five conditions, one of which entailed the use of disulfiram (Antabuse®). Since assignment to conditions was random, it was necessary to know in advance if an individual was going to be unwilling or medically unable to take disulfiram. Consequently, eligible individuals were asked about their willingness to take disulfiram, and those who refused were placed in track 2. Medical eligibility was determined by the project's physician upon completing a physical and examining laboratory results. Primary contraindications for disulfiram use were myocardial infarction, insulin-dependent diabetes mellitus, GGTP greater than 100 mU/mL, incapacitating organic disorder, and pregnancy. Medically ineligible participants also were placed in track 2.

The design and cell sizes were as follows. *Track 1 = willing and medically able to take disulfiram.* Within track 1 there were three conditions to which individuals were randomly assigned: CRA plus disulfiram ($n = 21$), CRA without disulfiram ($n = 19$), and standard treatment (STD; $n = 21$). *Track 2 = unwilling or medically unable to take disulfiram.* Track 2 consisted of random assignment to two groups: CRA without disulfiram ($n = 24$) and STD ($n = 21$). As noted, this design allowed us to address questions about possible motivational benefits associated with an individual's willingness to take disulfiram, and any disadvantages related to medical ineligibility. The present discussion will focus on the results for a simplified two-group design, in which the three CRA conditions were collapsed ($n = 64$) and contrasted with the two combined STD groups ($n = 42$).

CRA condition

A slightly modified version of CRA (Hunt & Azrin, 1973; Meyers & Smith, 1995) was used as the experimental condition. The assessment components of CRA were conducted during individual sessions, while the treatment was administered primarily in a group format. The former included the CRA Functional Analyses For Drinking and Nondrinking Behaviors, the Happiness Scale, and the Goals of Counseling plan. The one treatment procedure that was always conducted individually was sobriety sampling. Two behavioral skills training groups were offered daily, with the most common ones being problem-solving, drink refusal, and communication skills training. Additionally, specialized groups were offered occasionally in areas such as independent living skills. Also, each week started with a goal-setting group, in which individualized behavioral contracts were made for the upcoming week. Progress in these areas was checked and reinforced during a group meeting every Friday. The Social Club activity for the week was also decided during Friday's meeting. Typically the Social Club event was a leisurely dinner hosted by two of the CRA therapists at a local restaurant. One additional group was the disulfiram-compliance meeting, which was held each morning for all members of the CRA-plus-disulfiram condition. The nurse and the other group participants served as the crucial disulfiram monitors (Azrin, 1976; Azrin et al., 1982). Couples therapy was utilized with the few participants who had significant others. The final piece of the CRA program was the Job Club, which consisted of individualized assistance in job seeking (*see* Azrin & Besalel, 1982). The Job Club was open several hours each day.

The CRA therapists were advanced graduate students in clinical psychology who were behavioral in orientation. Their adherence to the treatment protocol was monitored through weekly supervision sessions and direct observation. With the exception of the Social Club, all treatment was delivered at the day shelter.

Standard treatment (STD)

Participants assigned to this condition were encouraged to take advantage of the many services regularly offered at the day shelter. These included sessions with a masters-level 12-step substance-abuse counselor, Alcoholics Anonymous (AA) meetings, a temporary job placement program, and case management meetings.

Treatment length and degree of participation were tailored to the individual. However, all CRA group members were required to attend groups regularly for the first 3 weeks of the program. At that point some individuals negotiated a new contract whereby they were allowed to work part-time during the day and attend only some of the normally recommended groups. At least minimal participation was required while individuals were living in the grant-sponsored housing. A CRA group member was considered a treatment drop-out if he or she attended less than 50% of the available groups during the first 3 weeks of their involvement in the program. Since there were no specific attendance requirements for the STD group participants, they could never be designated treatment drop-outs. The purpose of this design component was to test the day shelter's program as it was typically utilized.

Housing

Participants in both conditions were required to live in grant-supported apartments that housed two to four people. Individuals always lived with others in their same treatment condition. Although normally the length of stay was expected to be 3 months, individuals who had obtained a job and saved an agreed-upon amount of money were allowed to stay an extra month. Abstinence was required as a condition of housing. CRA participants had to take random breathalyzer tests, and offenders were suspended from the apartments for 1 week initially. To be allowed to return to the housing they had to attend CRA groups sober every day that week. Subsequent infractions carried 2-week suspensions. Although STD group participants were not regularly checked with breathalyzer tests, abstinence was expected, and they were suspended from housing temporarily if reports were received about their problematic behavior.

The results

Follow-up rates

Follow-up rates exceeded 75% for each of the five follow-up time periods, with rates declining from 93% at the initial 2-month follow-up to 76% at the final 12-month follow-up. A total of 78 subjects (74.6%) were located and assessed at all five follow-ups. Importantly, the average follow-up rates were virtually identical across the two conditions, with the difference being less than 1%.

Treatment effectiveness: drinking behavior

The three main dependent variables for assessing drinking behavior were: total number of drinks (standard ethanol content, SECs) per week, number of drinking days per week, and peak blood alcohol content (BAC) estimated from the steady drinking pattern reported (*see* Markham, Miller & Arciniega, 1993). Using the first of these measures, a participant was classified as abstinent at a given follow-up period if SECs consumed since the prior assessment was 0.

Preliminary tests of track and disulfiram effects

Preliminary tests indicated no evidence of the hypothesized potential benefits associated with being willing and able to take disulfiram, or with actually being assigned to take disulfiram. Thus, as noted previously, for the present chapter we will ignore the distinction between tracks and between disulfiram conditions, and will focus only on the comparison between CRA and STD.

Comparison of groups prior to treatment

As a check on the random assignment to conditions, tests for possible pretreatment differences between the CRA and STD groups were carried out. No differences were found on any intake measures of drinking behavior, on any of the demographic variables, on any of the intake liver enzyme measures, on willingness to take disulfiram, or on the proportion of participants who were dually diagnosed.

Treatment received

CRA participants attended an average of 39.3 CRA groups, 4.6 individual sessions, and 3.3 Job Club sessions. The only noteworthy individual variation across treatment components received was the Job Club training, in which 25% of participants did not attend any sessions, and 24% attended six or more times. The parts of the STD program that were considered the main treatment components were AA meetings, individual therapy sessions, and the day shelter's job program. The average number of AA meetings attended by the STD group members during the first 2 months of the program was 18.7. The number of documented individual sessions with the 12-step counselor averaged 0.8 sessions. However, the counselor reported that this was an underestimate, since many informal, unrecorded meetings were held with STD participants in various locations throughout the day shelter. The documentation for involvement in the day shelter's job program was also unavailable. In terms of overlap between treatments received in the STD and CRA groups, there was only one case of a CRA participant utilizing the 12-step counselor, and this occurred on three occasions. Although CRA participants did attend an average of 6.1 AA meetings during their treatment phase, this was significantly fewer than those attended by STD group members [$F(1,100) = 5.56, p = 0.0204$].

At each follow-up, participants were asked about additional help they had sought since the last assessment. In accordance with the Follow-up Drinker Profile's instructions, a score between 0 and 6 was assigned based on the number of categories of additional help sought. There were no differences across groups on this measure at any of the follow-up periods. On the other hand, the number of AA meetings that those in the STD group reported attending was higher than the number reported by CRA participants at each follow-up. But aside from the 2-month follow-up, the differences were not significant.

"Intention-to-treat" analysis

We first examined the question of primary interest by using all valid participants who were randomly assigned to conditions, including those who dropped out before receiving a sufficient dose of treatment. After summarizing overall tests using these 106 subjects, more fine-grained analyses are reported for the 101 treated subjects. While information from all five follow-ups was available for only 78 participants, 12 others had nearly complete information. Thus, to avoid eliminating participants because of missing data, an estimate of the missing data points for these 12 individuals was computed via linear regression based on their available follow-up information.

The change from intake to post-treatment averaging across all participants was dramatic on all three dependent variables. A multivariate test of change on these variables was highly significant [$F(3,98) = 58.77$, $p < 0.0001$], as were the separate univariate tests of change for number of drinks per week, drinking days per week, and steady-pattern peak BAC (all $ps < 0.0001$). Mean SECs per week declined from 136 per week before treatment to 22 post-treatment, mean drinking days declined from 5 to 1.4 days per week, and mean peak BAC declined from 287 mg% to 90 mg%.

The "intention-to-treat" analysis of the CRA effect also revealed significant results for the overall multivariate test and for all associated univariate tests. Group differences were assessed by MANCOVAs using as dependent variables the mean across the follow-ups for drinks per week post-treatment (note: a rank transformation was used because of the skewed distribution of the original SEC variable), drinking days per week post-treatment, and steady pattern peak BAC post-treatment. The intake values on the corresponding measures were used as covariates throughout, along with two variables from the BDP that were predictive of higher post-treatment drinking: frequency of other drug use and number of alcohol-related problems.

This summary MANCOVA of the difference between the CRA and STD conditions was significant even when drop-outs were included in the CRA condition with the multivariate $F(3,92) = 3.00$, $p = 0.0347$. The univariate tests were also significant, with $F(1,94) = 9.03$, $p = 0.0034$ for the SECs measure, $F(1, 94) = 6.19$, $p = 0.0146$ for drinking days per week, and $F(1,94) = 5.75$, $p = 0.0184$ for peak steady-pattern BAC. In each case the overall means indicated less drinking in the CRA condition than in the standard condition.

Analysis of "treated" participants

More detailed analyses examining effects at each follow-up time point were conducted using only those participants who received an adequate dose of treatment. This required eliminating only five subjects. MANCOVAs of the condition effect at each follow-up period were conducted on the basis of the observed data of whichever individuals were assessed at that time. In brief, there was a significant difference in favor of the CRA condition in either the multivariate test or one or more of the univariate tests at each of the follow-ups. The differences were quite consistent across the dependent variables at 2, 4, 6, and 9 months, with the multivariate F values being, respectively, $F(3,86) = 4.08$, $p = 0.0093$, $F(3,79) = 4.65$, $p = 0.0048$, $F(3,75) = 2.84$, $p = 0.0435$, and $F(3,75) = 4.19$, $p = 0.0085$. At 12 months,

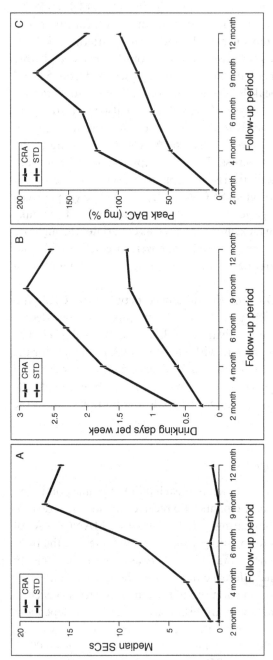

Figure 6.1 The Community Reinforcement Approach (CRA) group is contrasted with the standard treatment (STD) group at five follow-up times: on median standard ethanol content (SECs) per week, with one SEC representing one standard drink (A); on mean number of drinking days per week (B); and on the peak blood alcohol concentration (BAC) for the steady drinking pattern. From "The Community Reinforcement Approach with homeless alcohol-dependent individuals," by J. E. Smith, R. J. Meyers and H. D. Delaney, 1998, *Journal of Consulting and Clinical Psychology*, **66**, p.546. Copyright 1998 by the American Psychological Association, Inc. Reprinted with permission.

the multivariate test missed significance despite the fact that the univariate test of the treatment effect on drinks per week was still significant.

The average values of these variables for the CRA and STD conditions at each follow-up period are shown in Figure 6.1. As can be seen, the direction of the difference between groups favored the CRA condition on all three measures at all time points. The consistency of CRA's advantage was supported by the repeated-measures analyses performed separately on the three dependent variables, in which the test of the group by follow-up time period interaction yielded an F value of less than 1.0 in each case.

One slight exception to this consistency was in the greater than average difference between groups at 9 months and the less than average difference at 12 months. As seen in the figure, this seemed to be due to the fluctuation in the drinking levels of the STD group. A partial explanation may be the varying follow-up rates in this group.

Another way of measuring the effect of treatment on drinking behavior was to examine the proportion of participants who had been abstinent since the previous assessment. At the 2-month follow-up, the majority of participants tested (56%) reported being abstinent. Although this declined somewhat over time, at the 12-month follow-up a third of the tested individuals reported being abstinent. Group differences in abstinence rates, like the difference in the continuous drinking measures, were in favor of the CRA condition. These differences in rates were significant at 2 months [χ^2 $(1,N=95)=10.614$, $p=0.001$], at 4 months [χ^2 $(1,N=88)=8.47$, $p=0.004$], and at 9 months [χ^2 $(1,N=84)=7.16$, $p=0.007$].

Treatment effectiveness: additional drinking-related variables

The ASI and blood chemistry profiles were assessed pretreatment and again at the 6-month and 12-month follow-ups. Although group differences in these variables were not as pronounced as for the measures previously reported, they corroborated at least to some degree the benefits of CRA. For the ASI variable that reported the number of days of alcohol use in the past 30 days, there was a significant average decline from intake (11.7 days) to 6 months (6.3 days) [$t(79)=4.20$, $p<0.0001$]. Group differences at 6 months were not significant. However, the group difference at 12 months was significant in an ANCOVA test which covaried intake levels [$F(1,75)=4.73$, $p=0.033$], with the mean of 4.8 days in the CRA group being less than that of 9.9 days in the STD group.

Analyses of the blood chemistry profiles also generally showed mean differences favoring the CRA group, but only significantly so at the 6-month follow-up. We conducted ANCOVAs using the corresponding pretreatment liver enzyme levels as the covariate. Results at 6 months were significant for GGTP [$F(1,59) = 4.96$, $p = 0.0297$], with the CRA group's intake average (89.2 U/l) dropping down to within the normal range (53.0 U/l) and the STD group's intake level (67.5 U/l) increasing to an abnormally high level (107.3 U/l). The test for AST (SGOT) was marginal [$F(1,59) = 3.82$, $p = 0.0553$], with the CRA intake mean (45.2 U/l) remaining slightly elevated at 44.4 U/l, and the STD intake level (54.2 U/l) increasing to 84.9 U/l. For ALT (SGPT), the CRA intake mean of 55.0 U/l decreased to 45.5 U/l, whereas the STD intake average (65.3 U/l) increased to 97.3 U/l. This group difference was significant [$F(1,52) = 4.31$, $p = 0.043$], with the ALT values placing the CRA group within the normal range and the STD group in the elevated range.

Employment and housing outcomes

Employment and housing status improved markedly for both conditions throughout the project. The difference in rate of employment overall was highly significant when the rate at intake (9% employed) was compared with that at each follow-up period (all $p < 0.0001$). At 12 months the majority of the individuals (55%) for whom employment status was available had jobs. The change was confirmed by analyses of the ASI item giving number of days employed in the last 30. Whereas at intake participants reported a mean of 3.6 days employed, at 12 months the average was 10.9 days. Although this was a highly significant difference [$t(79) = 5.91$, $p < 0.0001$], there were no between-group differences in employment status at any time point.

Finally, there was also a clear decrease in the homelessness of study participants, with homelessness rates averaging less than 20% across the five follow-ups. In terms of group differences, the one statistically significant finding was at 4 months, when the rate of homelessness in the CRA group (13.7%) was lower than that in the STD (34%) [$\chi^2 (1, N = 86) = 5.10$, $p = 0.024$]. However, if one examines the subset of housed individuals who were actually paying for a more permanent type of dwelling at 12 months as opposed to just staying with friends or in a motel, the picture also favors the CRA group (62.5%) over the STD (44%) [$\chi^2 (1, N = 80) = 2.73$, $p < 0.10$].

The interpretation

Summary of alcohol findings

This study was a controlled comparison of CRA and a day shelter's standard treatment for alcohol-dependent homeless individuals. Dramatic reductions in drinking were found for both conditions, with the pretreatment mean of 19 drinks per day decreasing to 3.8 daily drinks at the 12-month follow-up. In contrasting the CRA and STD groups at this follow-up, the median number of daily drinks was 0.9 and 2.3, respectively. As noted, the CRA condition outperformed the STD on all three BDP drinking measures and across all follow-ups. Nevertheless, these between-group differences were less robust at the final follow-up. In part, we believe this was because our research assistants were unable to locate some of the STD group's heavier drinkers at this time; participants who were included in the noteworthy differences at 9 months.

The prediction that CRA group members who received disulfiram would consume significantly less alcohol than CRA participants within the same track who did not receive it was not supported. There are several possible explanations for this. First, we could argue that a floor effect was realized, given that each of the CRA conditions did extremely well. But the conclusion would still be that disulfiram was not necessary; that the CRA program without the disulfiram component was sufficient. This conclusion is contrary to the finding that disulfiram is a useful treatment adjunct with socially unstable clients (Azrin et al., 1982). However, one should also remember some of the unique parameters of the current study of homeless people, such as comfortable housing being available for individuals who could remain sober. It was also the case that individuals assigned to the CRA-plus-disulfiram condition only remained on the medication for approximately 5.5 weeks. So on average these individuals were off their disulfiram for at least several weeks before the first follow-up. Finally, the administration of disulfiram in the current study was different from that in other studies, inasmuch as the critical disulfiram monitors were the study's nurse and the other group members, as opposed to a loved one of the drinker (Azrin, 1976; Azrin et al., 1982). This was necessary, given the lack of available significant others for the participants. In sum, although the use of disulfiram in the present context did not contribute significantly to the positive outcome, one should be cautious in drawing conclusions about its utility in less controlled situations.

We also predicted that individuals who were both willing and medically eligible to take disulfiram would have an advantage over those who were not. This was based on the premise that the initial agreement to take disulfiram could be tapping a motivational factor, and that medical ineligibility implies a more serious alcohol problem. This prediction was not supported either. Furthermore, a motivational advantage was not detected when willingness to take disulfiram was examined separately from the eligibility factor. In order to interpret these findings one should first note the substantial discrepancy in expressed willingness to take disulfiram when comparing the first half of the sample recruited (52% willing) to the second half (87% willing). We had reason to suspect that participants being screened during the second half of the recruitment phase mistakenly believed that they had a greater likelihood of being accepted into the study if they reported during the intake that they were even willing to take disulfiram.

Summary of employment and housing findings

With regard to the nondrinking outcomes, both groups showed improvements. The pretreatment employment rate of 9% increased to 55% at the time of the 12-month follow-up. This still left 45% of the total sample unemployed. Furthermore, among those who were working, only 23% of them were in full-time positions. Another way of looking at the outcome is in terms of the number of days employed in the last 30. The average number of days at intake was 3.6, while the mean at 12 months was 10.9 days. These findings are quite similar to those found in several earlier studies of the homeless (Braucht et al., 1995; Lapham et al., 1995), and much better than others (NIAAA, 1992b; Toro et al., 1997).

These modest changes in employment status merit investigation, as there appears to be much room for improvement. Additionally, there are those who believe that chronic unemployment plays a major role in limiting the long-term success of substance-abuse treatment programs (Platt, 1995). Along with economic security, employment is credited with providing enhanced self-confidence and social functioning, and is associated with decreases in both criminality and substance abuse (Joe, Chastain & Simpson, 1990; Schottenfeld, Pascale & Sokolowski, 1992). In examining the employment issue in the current study, we believe that one critical piece of the problem was the fact that attendance at the job program for either condition was poor. As far as CRA's Job Club, since it was "open" every weekday, there were 40 possible sessions during an individual's first 2 months in the program. However, participants attended it an average of only 3.3 times. When we encouraged participants to take advantage of the Job Club, they informed us that they did not really need it because they knew how to get a job. While this was certainly the case for many, the jobs they obtained were often ones that either placed them at risk of relapse, or proved to be aversive in relatively short periods of time. Future studies will need to explore ways to motivate individuals to utilize job finding services, and perhaps job skills training (Brewington et al., 1987).

In terms of homelessness status, there was an overall dramatic decrease from the 100% pretreatment rate to the less than 15% rate at 12 months. In part, this improvement may have resulted indirectly from the substantial reductions in alcohol use, since many were then welcomed back into the homes of loved ones. But certainly as employment rates increased, the ability to finance a dwelling increased as well. Additionally, the grant offered an incentive of a fourth month of free housing for those who had a job and had saved an agreed-upon amount of money at the end of their 3 months in the apartments. Many participants in both conditions utilized this offer. As far as between-group differences, the CRA condition showed a slight advantage at all but the 6-month follow-up, but the only significant difference was at 4 months. This advantage was even more pronounced when we compared only those individuals who were living in more permanent types of dwellings as opposed to staying in hotels or with friends.

Limitations of the study

Since the study was designed as a comparison between CRA and a day shelter's standard program as it was typically used, equal doses of treatment were not contrasted. A large variety of substance-abuse services were available at the shelter, and yet many of the STD participants chose not to rely on them. In fact, we learned that they nicknamed their condition the "independent study" group, signifying their belief that they should get back on track on their own during the time that they were being given free living accommodations. It was also the case that although abstinence was required of all participants while living in the grant-supported housing, routine breathalyzer tests were only conducted on CRA group members as part of their behavioral contingencies. The role that this played in the positive treatment outcome is unknown.

An additional limitation of the study was the fact that some self-selection occurred. As noted, 213 potential participants initially inquired about the program, but 67 of them disappeared either immediately upon reading the consent form or somewhere midway through the intake assessment. It is our belief that once the requirements of the program (i.e., staying sober and getting a job) became clear during the course of intake, many individuals decided that they were unwilling to alter their behavior in exchange for free housing. However, it is possible that a number of motivated individuals simply felt unable to comply with these requirements. A final limitation of the study is the cost of treatment. Although the CRA program is generally considered one of the most cost-effective alcohol treatments (Finney & Monahan, 1996), this version of CRA included an expensive new component: housing. However, since many homeless agencies today have transitional housing programs in place, it is conceivable that these agencies could make housing arrangements for participants in a CRA treatment program, thereby keeping the cost down.

Future research

This study was the first test of CRA with a homeless population. The promising results were obtained while using a cost-effective group format by relatively inexperienced therapists. Additionally, the low drop-out and high follow-up rates ensure that the findings were representative of the sample in general, and they also bode well for successfully conducting future research with this approach. One question that remains is how to prevent the gradual rise in drinking levels that was evident across the follow-up period. A second question is how to better address the needs of the subset of CRA group participants (approximately 10%) who were virtually treatment nonresponders. Furthermore, changes need to be made to increase attendance at the job finding program. In conjunction with this, the program should also offer a job skills training component, and should then take steps to ensure that individuals participate in it. Finally, the small number of women in the project precluded a comparison of their outcomes in the CRA and STD programs. Future studies should focus on women's responses to the CRA program so that the necessary adaptations can be instituted.

7

CRA and Treatment of Cocaine and Opioid Dependence

STEPHEN T. HIGGINS AND PATRICK J. ABBOTT

In this chapter we review research on use of the Community Reinforcement Approach (CRA) in outpatient treatment for cocaine and opioid dependence. Briefly, CRA is a multicomponent behavioral treatment that was originally developed for the treatment of alcoholism (Hunt & Azrin, 1973). CRA is designed to systematically facilitate changes in the client's daily environment to reduce substance abuse and promote a healthier lifestyle. Systematic efforts are made to increase the frequency and amount of reinforcement clients derive from their vocation, family relations, and social and recreational activities so that those areas might compete more successfully with the allure of the pharmacological and social reinforcement obtained through substance abuse. The treatment also involves skills training tailored to meet individual needs, including skills directly related to decreasing substance use (e.g., functional analysis of drug use, drug refusal training) and others important to increasing reinforcement derived from a healthier lifestyle (e.g., problem solving, social skills training, sleep-hygiene training). Treatment duration can vary from 2 to 6 months, and usually involves up to several individual therapy sessions weekly delivered by professional therapists trained in this treatment approach. CRA can also be delivered in group sessions (Azrin, 1976). Those interested in a more detailed description of CRA or information on clinical implementation should consult Chapters 1 and 3 of this volume and the published therapy manuals (Budney & Higgins, 1998; Meyers & Smith, 1995).

Effective psychosocial interventions like CRA are fundamentally important to the treatment of cocaine and opioid dependence. Psychosocial interventions are the only treatments demonstrated to be reliably efficacious with cocaine-dependent individuals (Higgins & Wong, 1998). Effective pharmacological treatments for cocaine dependence have not yet been identified, although, as is discussed below, monitored disulfiram therapy appears to be effective with individuals concurrently dependent on cocaine and alcohol (Carroll et al., 1998). Several efficacious pharmacological treatments for opioid dependence are available, but outcomes are improved substantially when those medications are combined with efficacious psychosocial interventions like CRA (McLellan et al., 1993; Onken, Blaine & Boren, 1995).

CRA in the treatment of cocaine dependence

Cocaine abuse remains a major public health problem in the United States that contributes to many of our most disturbing individual and societal problems. Cocaine abuse contributes to increased crime and incarceration, psychopathology, drug-exposed neonates, the spread of acquired immune deficiency disorder (AIDS), tuberculosis (TB), hepatitis and other infectious diseases, poverty, trauma, and violence (Konkol & Olsen, 1996; Montoya & Atkinson, 1996; National Institute of Justice, 1999; Substance Abuse and Mental Health Services Administration, 1997a–c; Tardiff et al., 1994). While progress has been made in reducing the overall size of the U.S. cocaine-abuse epidemic, major problems remain. In a recent National Household Survey, for example, 2.6 million members of U.S. households aged 12 years and older reported using cocaine in the past year, 1.5 million reported use in the past month, and 682,000 reported using once a week or more (Substance Abuse and Mental Health Services Administration, 1997a–c). While the 2.6 million estimate represents a 65% reduction from the estimated 7.1 million past-year users reported in 1985, the estimates for past-month and weekly users have remained stable since 1992 and 1985, respectively (Substance Abuse and Mental Health Services Administration, 1998). This stable, core group of heavy cocaine users accounts for most of the problems associated with cocaine abuse, and is the group for whom effective treatments are sorely needed.

As is noted above, more progress has been made in the development of efficacious psychosocial than pharmacological treatments for cocaine dependence. One of those efficacious psychosocial treatments is an intervention that combines CRA with a voucher-based incentive program. Before describing the research that supports the efficacy of this treatment, a brief description of the rationale for adding the voucher-based incentives to CRA is warranted. In developing this treatment for cocaine dependence in the late 1980s, the goal was to develop an intervention to treat cocaine dependence in outpatient settings. One of the major challenges of out-patient treatment of cocaine dependence is the high rates of early attrition (Higgins & Budney, 1997). Attrition rates of 50–75% within the first few weeks of outpatient treatment are common. A clinic-based incentive pro-gram involving material reinforcers was deemed a potentially cost-effective alternative to hospitalization for retaining these individuals in treatment. Another major concern when putting this treatment together was how to compete early in the treatment process with the powerful reinforcing effects of cocaine use. Time is needed to bring about sufficient lifestyle changes so that a sober lifestyle might offer sufficient naturalistic reinforce-ment to compete effectively with the reinforcing effects of cocaine use. The incentive program was conceived as a means of having an effective re-inforcer for cocaine abstinence in place during the initial phases of treat-ment, and to thereby gain the time needed to implement the more familiar aspects of CRA so that effective naturalistic alternatives would be avail-able later to help sustain longer-term abstinence. Said differently, the goal was to use a relatively contrived reinforcement system for abstinence early in treatment and then to help the clients' transition to a more naturalistic system of reinforcement for abstinence during the later part of treatment and aftercare. It is worth emphasizing that cocaine abstinence is the goal of this treatment approach, but problems with ongoing drug use and relapse are expected and handled as a normal part of the treatment process.

Seminal clinical trials

Two clinical trials provided the initial empirical evidence supporting the efficacy of the CRA plus vouchers treatment (Higgins et al., 1991, 1993*b*). Both involved comparisons to standard outpatient drug-abuse counseling. The first of these two trials was 12 weeks in duration and 28 clients were assigned to the respective treatment groups as consecutive clinic admis-sions, while the second trial involved 24 weeks of treatment and 38 clients were assigned randomly to the two treatment groups. In both trials the CRA plus vouchers treatment retained clients in treatment significantly longer than standard counseling and resulted in significantly longer per-iods of documented cocaine abstinence. For example, in the randomized trial, 58% of patients assigned to the CRA plus vouchers treatment com-pleted 24 weeks of treatment versus 11% of those assigned to standard counseling. Furthermore, 68% and 42% of patients in the CRA plus vouchers group were documented to have achieved 8 and 16 weeks of continuous cocaine abstinence versus 11% and 5% of those in the counseling group (Figure 7.1). Follow-up assessments were conducted at 9 and 12 months after treatment entry in the randomized trial (Higgins et al., 1995). Significantly greater cocaine abstinence was documented through urinalysis at the 9- and 12-month follow-ups in the CRA plus vouchers group than the standard counseling group, while both groups showed comparable and significant improvements on the Addiction Severity Index (ASI) (McLellan, Luborsky & Cacciola, 1985). This pattern of discerning relatively robust treatment differences in retention and abstinence, but generally not in other areas of functioning, is a consistent finding across many of the trials reviewed in this chapter.

These two trials provided some of the earliest and most definitive scientific evidence that cocaine dependence could indeed be managed effectively in outpatient settings. Outpatient treatment has now become the norm for treating cocaine dependence, except in cases of special medical circumstances or when individuals repeatedly fail to make any clinically significant progress in reducing their cocaine use during outpatient care (Higgins & Wong, 1998).

Research efforts with this treatment approach next turned to examining the efficacy of particular components of the multielement intervention. This practice of experimentally dismantling the treatment can help to streamline the intervention by eliminating ineffective elements, and can also identify effective components for potential dissemination separate from the rest of the treatment. Both have resulted from the research described below.

Monitored disulfiram therapy

The benefits of CRA's origins in the treatment of alcohol dependence came to the forefront early in its use with the cocaine-dependent population. Sixty percent or more of individuals presenting for treatment for cocaine dependence may meet the diagnostic criteria for alcohol dependence (Higgins et al., 1994b). Monitored disulfiram therapy is a major component of CRA for the treatment of alcohol problems (see Chapters 1 and 3, this volume) and thus was adopted as part of the CRA plus vouchers treatment for cocaine dependence and offered to all individuals who reported evidence of concurrent alcohol dependence or noted a direct relationship between their alcohol and cocaine use. The original intent was to use monitored disulfiram therapy for the sole purpose of treating the

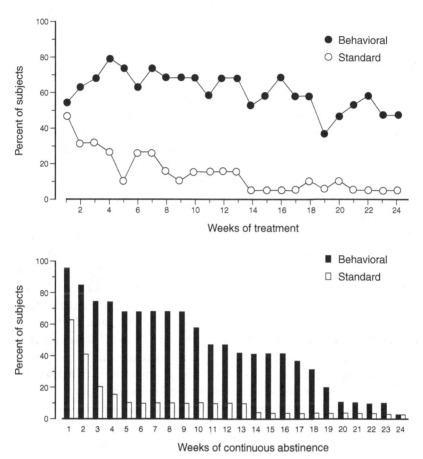

Figure 7.1 Upper panel: percent of subjects abstinent during consecutive treatment weeks are shown for the Community Reinforcement Approach (CRA) (behavioral, filled symbols) and drug-abuse counseling (standard, unfilled symbols). Lower panel: the height of each bar indicates the percentage of subjects in each treatment group who achieved a duration of continuous cocaine abstinence equal to or greater than the number of weeks indicated. Note that the weeks of continuous abstinence could occur anywhere within the 24-week treatment. Symbols are the same as in the upper panel. Reprinted with permission from Higgins et al., 1993*b*.

alcohol problems, but as the practice was researched it was learned that it also reduced cocaine use. The term monitored is used here to denote that clinic staff and significant others were used to monitor and support compliance with the recommended medication regimen. Such support for compliance with the recommended dosing regimen appears to be necessary for disulfiram therapy to be effective (Azrin et al., 1982). Even with support strategies in place, sustaining compliance with disulfiram is often an ongoing clinical challenge.

As a first step toward assessing the contribution of the disulfiram element of this CRA plus vouchers treatment to outcome, a chart review was conducted with 16 individuals who met DSM III-R criteria for cocaine dependence and alcohol abuse/dependence (Higgins et al., 1993a). Subjects were chosen on the basis of having at least 2 weeks on and off disulfiram therapy (usually 250 mg daily), which permitted an opportunity to assess for associated benefits. Both drinking and cocaine-positive urinalysis results were more than twofold lower while on versus off disulfiram therapy in this chart review.

The uncontrolled nature of the chart-review study precluded causal inferences to be drawn regarding the contribution of disulfiram therapy to the observed reductions in cocaine use. However, the findings from that uncontrolled study were supported by results from two randomized trials that did permit causal inferences to be made. Note that in these trials monitored disulfiram therapy was divorced from CRA and delivered in combination with other psychosocial interventions. Carroll and colleagues (Carroll et al., 1993) reported results from a pilot trial in which 18 outpatients being treated for alcohol and cocaine abuse were randomized to receive disulfiram or naltrexone therapy in combination with interpersonal psychotherapy. Disulfiram therapy resulted in threefold or greater reductions in drinking and cocaine use than naltrexone therapy. While those effects were encouraging, the number of subjects was small and there was considerable attrition.

To investigate further the possible efficacy of disulfiram therapy, a larger randomized trial was completed with 120 outpatients with concurrent cocaine and alcohol dependence or abuse (Carroll et al., 1998). Individuals were randomized to one of five treatment groups: cognitive behavior therapy (CBT) alone or with monitored disulfiram therapy (CBT/Disulf), 12-step facilitation (TSF) therapy alone or with monitored disulfiram therapy (TSF/Disulf), and clinical management plus monitored disulfiram (CM/Disulf). CM is a minimal intervention that had been used as a control condition in prior trials examining the efficacy of relapse prevention in the treatment of cocaine dependence. Disulfiram therapy significantly increased mean weeks of retention, and there was no interaction with the type of psychosocial treatment. Additionally, patients who received disulfiram achieved significantly more consecutive weeks of cocaine abstinence, alcohol abstinence, and cocaine plus alcohol abstinence compared to patients who received no medication, with no significant interactions between medication and type of psychotherapy (Table 7.1). These promising positive results achieved with disulfiram stand in stark contrast to the negative results that have been observed with almost all of the other pharmacotherapies for cocaine dependence tested to date (Mendelson & Mello, 1996).

Relationship counseling

When the CRA plus vouchers treatment was initially developed, there was a component in which clients were encouraged to include a significant other (SO) in the treatment process. If available, preference was for a wife, husband, or other romantic partner who was not a substance abuser. If a romantic partner was not available, clients were encouraged to involve anyone who was not a substance abuser and was sincerely interested in their success in treatment. SOs and clients were taught to develop behavioral contracts wherein clients agreed to maintain cocaine abstinence and the SOs agreed to do something positive for clients (e.g., go out to lunch) when urinalysis results were cocaine-negative. When romantic partners were involved, behavioral relationship counseling was provided as well. A retrospective analysis conducted with 52 cocaine-dependent individuals who had received this intervention as part of the CRA plus vouchers treatment indicated that including an SO in treatment was a robust predictor of a positive treatment outcome (Higgins et al., 1994*a*). There were no differences between romantic and nonromantic partners in that regard, suggesting that the important variable was the SO–client contract around urinalysis results and not the relationship counseling provided to those with romantic partners. To follow-up on this interesting correlation, a randomized trial was conducted in which 58 cocaine-dependent clients were randomized to the usual CRA plus vouchers treatment or to CRA plus vouchers minus the SO component (Higgins et al., 1994*a*). Including an SO in treatment had no discernible effects on treatment retention, cocaine abstinence, or any other outcome measure in that trial (not shown). Thus, these results suggested that while those individuals in the earlier trials who included SOs in their treatment had better outcomes, this was probably not a causal relationship. Hence, the practice of teaching clients and SOs to develop behavioral contracts regarding urinalysis

Table 7.1. *Rates of consecutive abstinence by treatment, n=117*

	Treatment condition					Significance of effect		
	TSF $n=23$	CBT $n=18$	CM/Disulf $n=27$	TSF/Disulf $n=25$	CBT/Disulf $n=24$	Medication F, p	Psychotherapy F, p	Interaction
Maximum weeks of consecutive abstinence during treatment, mean (SD)								
Cocaine	2.22 (3.02)	1.83 (2.03)	2.59 (3.74)	3.76 (3.84)	4.54 (4.51)	7.67/0.007	3.80/0.05	NS
Alcohol	2.13 (3.36	1.27 (1.17)	3.85 (3.65)	4.92 (4.44)	4.62 (4.73)	14.38/0.000	1.12/0.29	NS
Both	1.82 (2.75)	1.05 (0.93)	2.00 (3.27)	3.72 (3.85)	3.50 (4.23)	9.49/0.003	4.02/0.04	NS
Number (%) of subjects achieving 3 or more weeks of consecutive abstinence during treatment								
Cocaine	7 (30.4%)	5 (21.7%)	8 (29.6%)	13 (52.0%)	14 (58.3%)	3.12/0.07	NS	NS
Alcohol	5 (21.7)	2 (15.4)	13 (48.1)	15 (60.0)	13 (54.2)	14.96/0.000	NS	NS
Both	5 (21.7)	1 (5.6)	6 (22.2)	12 (48.0)	11 (45.8)	7.02/0.008	NS	NS

TSF, 12-step facilitation; CBT, cognitive behavioral therapies; CB, clinical management. Medication effect reflects disulfiram–no disulfiram contrast. Psychotherapy comparison reflects comparison of CBT and TSF (active psychotherapies) to CM. Interaction indicates CBT/TSF by disulfiram/no medication. Reprinted from Carroll et al., 1998, with permission from Taylor & Francis, Oxfordshire, UK, http://www.tandf.co.uk/journals.

results was eliminated from the CRA plus vouchers treatment. That trial was not designed to assess the efficacy of the behavioral relationship counseling component and hence that service continues to be offered as part of this treatment. The positive improvements in relationship satisfaction and drug use that have been reported in other trials using behavioral relationship counseling with illicit substance abusers, including cocaine abusers, provide empirical support for retaining that component in the CRA plus vouchers treatment (Fals-Stewart, Birchler & O'Farrell, 1996).

Voucher-based incentives

Next, the contribution of the voucher-based incentive program to the positive outcomes achieved with this treatment was investigated in a series of randomized trials. The voucher system is in effect during weeks 1–12 of this 24-week CRA plus vouchers intervention. Clients earn vouchers for cocaine-negative urine toxicology test results under a Monday, Wednesday, and Friday monitoring schedule. The value of the vouchers increases with each consecutive cocaine-negative specimen delivered, and cocaine-positive specimens reset the value of vouchers back to their initial level. Those who are continuously abstinent throughout the 12-week voucher period can earn the equivalent of $973.50 in purchasing power. No cash is ever given to clients, and all voucher purchases are made by clinic staff who retain veto power over all requests and only approve them if they are in concert with the healthier lifestyle that the treatment is intended to promote.

In the first randomized trial examining the efficacy of this voucher program, 40 patients were assigned to receive CRA plus vouchers or CRA alone (Higgins et al., 1994c). Treatment was 24 weeks in duration and the voucher versus no-voucher difference was in effect during weeks 1–12 only. Both treatment groups were treated in the same way after week 12. Seventy-five percent of patients in the group with vouchers completed 24 weeks of treatment versus 40% in the CRA-alone group. The average duration of continuous cocaine abstinence documented through urinalysis in the two groups was 11.7±2.0 weeks in the vouchers group as opposed to 6.0 ± 1.5 in the no-vouchers group (Figure 7.2). At the end of the 24-week treatment period, significant decreases from pretreatment scores were observed in both treatment groups on the ASI family/social and alcohol scales, with no differences between the groups. Both groups

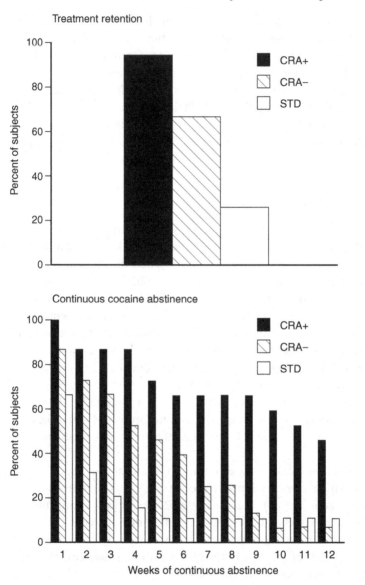

Figure 7.2 Upper panel: percent of subjects who completed at least 12 weeks of treatment when treated with CRA plus vouchers (CRA+, filled bars), CRA without vouchers (CRA−, striped bars), and drug-abuse counseling (STD, unfilled bars). Lower panel: the height of each bar indicates the percentage of subjects in each treatment group who achieved a duration of continuous cocaine abstinence equal to or greater than the number of weeks indicated. Note that the weeks of continuous abstinence could occur anywhere within the 12-week treatment period. Symbols are the same as in upper panel.

also decreased on the ASI drug scale, but the magnitude of change was significantly greater in the voucher than the no-voucher groups, and only the voucher group showed a significant improvement on the ASI psychiatric scale. These ASI results remained the same at the follow-up assessments completed 9 and 12 months after treatment entry (Higgins et al., 1995). These results provided compelling evidence regarding the contribution of the voucher component to the positive outcomes achieved previously with the CRA plus vouchers treatment.

While the results from this trial provided definitive evidence regarding the efficacy of the voucher component of this multielement treatment, they also provided an opportunity to contrast the results from the CRA plus vouchers and CRA-only groups in this trial with results obtained from the 19 subjects who received drug-abuse counseling in the randomized trial described above. Retention rates and documented levels of cocaine abstinence varied in a graded manner, with clients who received CRA plus vouchers having the best outcomes, those who received CRA alone somewhat poorer outcomes, and those who received drug-abuse counseling having the poorest outcomes (Figure 7.3). Note that these differences were observed in the absence of any discernible differences in the intake characteristics of the subjects treated. Such comparisons across trials must be interpreted cautiously, but the results observed with the CRA-alone group were consistent with a position that this treatment included active elements in addition to the vouchers. The evidence reviewed above on monitored disulfiram therapy and elsewhere in this chapter are consistent with that conclusion.

A recent trial on CRA plus vouchers provided an opportunity to assess the effects of contingent vouchers on cocaine abstinence separate from their effects on treatment retention (Higgins et al., 2000). This trial also extended follow-up assessments out to 1 year after completion of the 24-week CRA plus vouchers treatment and to 15 months after cessation of the voucher intervention. In prior trials, subjects who had received contingent vouchers had been retained in treatment for longer and had achieved greater cocaine abstinence than those in the comparison treatments. While they formed a very important outcome in themselves, the retention differences observed in those trials obscured interpretation of the mechanism of action. That is, the retention differences between the treatment groups made it difficult to dissociate the direct reinforcing effects of contingent incentives on cocaine abstinence from the indirect effects that may have arisen from a greater duration of counseling.

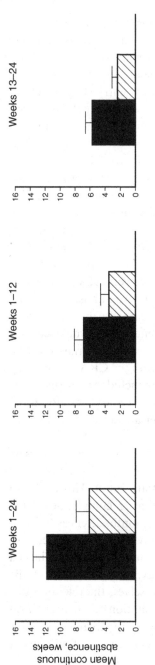

Figure 7.3 Mean duration of continuous cocaine abstinence documented through urinalysis testing in each treatment group during weeks 1–24 (entire treatment), 1–12 (voucher phase), and 13–24 (after vouchers ended) of treatment. Solid and shaded bars indicate CRA with vouchers and CRA without vouchers groups, respectively. Error bars represent ± SEM. Reprinted with permission from Higgins et al., 1994c.

To experimentally examine this matter, 70 cocaine-dependent adults were randomly assigned to receive CRA plus vouchers contingent on cocaine abstinence or CRA plus vouchers delivered independent of urinalysis results. The intention of making vouchers available to both treatment groups was to keep retention rates comparable between them. Making voucher availability contingent on cocaine-negative urinalysis results in one group but not the other permitted experimental isolation of the contribution of contingent reinforcement to cocaine abstinence.

As intended, there were no significant differences in treatment retention rates, or follow-up rates, between the two treatment groups. Nevertheless, cocaine abstinence differed significantly between the two groups, with, for example, threefold more subjects (36% versus 12%) in the contingent than the noncontingent groups achieving 12 or more weeks of continuous cocaine abstinence during treatment. Moreover, the point prevalence of cocaine abstinence at the end of treatment and at each of the follow-up assessments conducted 9, 12, 15, and 18 months after treatment entry was greater in the contingent group than in the noncontingent group (average difference = 16%). Those results demonstrate that contingent vouchers are capable of directly reinforcing cocaine abstinence and that those effects can remain discernible for up to 12 months following the end of the CRA plus vouchers treatment and for up to 15 months following the end of the contingent voucher component of that intervention.

Most of the research with CRA plus vouchers was conducted in rural Burlington, Vermont, which has an almost exclusively Caucasian population. Hence, an important question about those findings was whether they could be generalized to cocaine abusers in the inner-city and more ethnically diverse populations. To begin to address that matter, a controlled trial was completed examining the efficacy of the voucher program described above with cocaine-abusing methadone-maintenance patients in a clinic located in Baltimore, MD (Silverman et al., 1996a). As is described below, methadone is a medication used to treat heroin dependence (Ball & Ross, 1991). While very effective for heroin, it does not treat other concurrent drug-abuse problems such as cocaine abuse that are common in these patients. During a 12-week study, subjects in the experimental group ($n = 19$) received vouchers exchangeable for retail items contingent on cocaine-negative urinalysis tests. A matched control group ($n = 18$) received the vouchers independent of urinalysis results and according to a schedule that was yoked to the experimental group. Both groups received a standard form of outpatient drug-abuse counseling routinely offered to

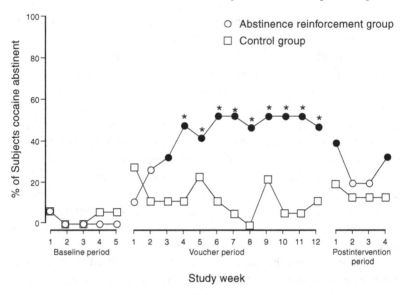

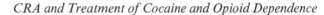

Figure 7.4 Percentage of patients abstinent during 25 successive study weeks. A patient was considered cocaine abstinent for a given week if all of the three urine samples for that week were negative for cocaine. Solid circles and asterisks indicate the weeks on which the abstinence reinforcement group value differed significantly from the control group value according to planned comparisons based on a repeated-measures analysis of variance ($p \leqslant 0.05$ and $p \leqslant 0.01$, respectively). Data for the 4-week postintervention period are based on the urinalysis results from subjects who completed the entire 4-week postintervention period (15 control and 15 abstinence reinforcement subjects). Reprinted with permission from Silverman et al., 1996*a*.

methadone-maintenance patients. Note that, like the monitored disulfiram component discussed above, the voucher program was investigated independent of the other CRA elements. Cocaine use was substantially reduced in the experimental group, but remained relatively unchanged in the control group (Figure 7.4). Both treatment groups were followed for 1 month following termination of the voucher intervention. Abstinence decreased in the contingent group compared to levels observed during the intervention period, but remained significantly above levels observed in the control group during weeks 1 and 4 of that 1 month of follow-up. Subsequent trials conducted at that same Baltimore site as well as other clinics located in other large metropolitan areas in the U.S. have further supported the efficacy of the voucher program with inner-city cocaine-dependent individuals (Rawson et al., 1999; Silverman et al., 1998). An additional finding from those trials merits mention. In several of the trials in which the voucher intervention was used to reduce cocaine use among methadone-maintenance patients, significant reductions in opioid use were found as well even though the abstinence contingency was specific to cocaine use (Silverman et al., 1996*a*, 1998). It is not yet fully understood why this occurs. It may result from decreasing the frequency of "speedballing" (i.e., simultaneous injection of cocaine and heroin mixtures) or alternatively perhaps subjects abstain from heroin use as a means of increasing the probability that they will succeed in their efforts to abstain from cocaine use.

Relationship between early and longer-term abstinence

Recently a study was conducted to further understand the predictors of longer-term cocaine abstinence (Higgins, Badger & Budney, 2000). During-treatment and post-treatment results were examined from 190 cocaine-dependent patients who participated in the clinical trials involving CRA plus vouchers described above. Subjects were divided into two groups: those treated with CRA plus contingent vouchers and those treated with one of the comparison treatments. The single best predictor of abstinence during follow-up for subjects treated with CRA plus vouchers or the comparison treatments was the amount of abstinence achieved during treatment. To provide a concrete example, among subjects treated with CRA plus vouchers who achieved at least 12 weeks of continuous abstinence during treatment, 41% were abstinent at each assessment throughout 6 months of post-treatment follow-up versus only 9% of those who achieved less during-treatment abstinence. Similar figures for those in the control treatments were 44% and 7% for those who did and did not achieve 12 or more weeks of during-treatment abstinence, respectively. There was no evidence of a threshold amount of during-treatment abstinence necessary for this relationship to become evident. Instead, the probability of post-treatment abstinence increased as an orderly, graded function of the amount of during-treatment abstinence achieved. One important difference between the CRA plus vouchers and comparison treatments with regard to this relationship was that a greater percentage of subjects in the former than the latter achieved sustained periods of cocaine abstinence during treatment and hence a larger percentage of them were abstinent during follow-up as well. Said differently, the prognostic significance of during-treatment abstinence was comparable between the CRA plus contingent vouchers and comparison treatments, but, because the CRA plus vouchers treatment promoted long periods of sustained abstinence during treatment in a larger percentage of clients than did the comparison treatments, it also produced greater abstinence during follow-up.

An important aspect of these findings is that they suggest that abstinence-contingent vouchers delivered in the context of CRA do not inflate abstinence levels while the incentives are in place only to see those effects dissipate precipitously when the vouchers are discontinued. Rather, the increased abstinence achieved during treatment with the contingent vouchers appears to have the same degree of longer-term benefit as abstinence achieved in the context of other treatments. These results contradict the notion that is sometimes fostered in substance-abuse treatment circles that early abstinence is not important and later abstinence is what clinicians should focus upon. Rather, these results suggest that during-treatment abstinence may be critically important and that, within the range of treatments examined, interventions that produce more during-treatment cocaine abstinence are also more likely to produce greater longer-term cocaine abstinence. Note that only outpatient treatments were included in this study. Whether abstinence achieved in the context of residential treatment or other protected environments has similar prognostic significance is an empirical question that is not addressed by this study.

Some ongoing research

A randomized trial is currently underway in Burlington, VT, examining the effects of CRA plus vouchers versus vouchers in combination with only very minimal support services. This trial is designed to isolate the contribution of CRA as a complete treatment package over and above the effects produced by contingent vouchers alone. It is too early to report results from that trial, which is approximately at the half-way point. Many other trials are ongoing nationally examining various applications of the vouchers component of the CRA plus vouchers treatment (e.g., see Higgins & Silverman, 1999), and Carroll and colleagues are continuing to research the use of disulfiram therapy with cocaine-dependent individuals (Carroll, 1999).

Treatment of opioid dependence

Numerous countries and cities from around the world have reported an increase in heroin availability and use (NIDA Notes, 1998). One of the main reasons for this is the increase of worldwide production and purity, which has resulted in reductions in the price of heroin. From 1992 to 1996, the world production of opium increased by approximately 1000 tons to a total of 4570 tons, which converts to approximately 450 tons of heroin (Cowell, 1997). The purity of heroin in the Northeastern U.S., for example, has increased to as high as 90%, which has contributed to a shift in the route of heroin administration from primarily injection to smoking or snorting.

Several recent national surveys have documented the rise of heroin use in the U.S., including the Drug Abuse Warning Network (DAWN), the National Household Survey on Drug Abuse, and the Monitoring the Futures Study. Heroin-related emergency department episodes rose from 33,900 in 1990 to 70,500 in 1996 with some leveling off in 1997 (Substance Abuse and Mental Health Services Administration, 1997*a–c*). This represents a doubling of heroin-related episodes from 15/100,000 to 30/100,000. The National Household Survey on Drug Abuse noted a fivefold increase in reported use of heroin between 1995 and 1996, with the majority of use occurring among individuals over the age of 35 and among males (Substance Abuse and Mental Health Services Administration, 1997*b*). Heroin use has increased in prevalence among high-school students, college students, and young adults (Johnston, O'Malley & Bachman, 1997). Additionally, heroin use has increased in 17 of the 21 Community Epidemiology Work Group (CEWG) areas in the U.S. in 1995 and 1996 (NIDA Notes, 1998). These studies note a rise in heroin use by youths from all socioeconomic classes, with a notable rise in middle-class youths (Stine & Kosten, 1997). The Monitoring the Futures Study also noted that a substantial percentage of recent heroin users are using by routes other than injection and that the "perceived risk" of use decreased in 1995 (Johnston, O'Malley & Bachman, 1997).

As expected, such increases in the prevalence of heroin use are associated with increases in heroin-related mortality and morbidity. Although the death rate from AIDS has slowed, a higher proportion of new cases of AIDS can be attributed to injection drug use (Holmberg, 1996). There is also the growing concern about the high prevalence among injection drug abusers of hepatitis B (HBC) and C (HCV), with HBC exceeding 60% and HCV 80% among many groups of injection drug users (Stine & Kosten, 1997).

CRA in the treatment of opioid dependence

Considering such increases in heroin availability, the prevalence of use, and heroin-related mortality and morbidity, the need for effective treatments for opioid dependence is clear. As was noted above, methadone, buprenorphine, and other pharmacotherapies are effective treatments for opioid dependence, but their efficacy is enhanced when combined with effective psychosocial interventions (Onken, Blaine & Boren, 1995). We know of two controlled trials demonstrating enhanced efficacy when CRA was used in combination with an effective pharmacotherapy, and one demonstrating the same with the voucher-based incentive program alone. One study was conducted in the context of a detoxification protocol (Bickel et al., 1997) and the others in the context of a maintenance protocol (Abbott et al., 1998*b*; Silverman et al., 1996*b*). In detoxification and maintenance protocols, physically dependent clients receive a prescription medication that substitutes pharmacologically for heroin, thereby reducing or preventing withdrawal symptomatology. In the detoxification protocol, the dose of the medication is gradually decreased over days, weeks, or months with the goal of having the client opioid free and without pronounced withdrawal symptomatology at the end of treatment. In the maintenance protocol, the goal is to stabilize and then maintain clients for an indefinite period of time on a dose of medication that prevents pronounced withdrawal and decreases or eliminates use of heroin and other illicit opioids.

Detoxification study

Unfortunately, opioid detoxification protocols are noted for their lack of efficacy (e.g., Bickel et al., 1988). Typically retention and abstinence rates are clinically reasonable early in the detoxification while the dose of medication is still relatively high, and then they fall off precipitously as the medication dose is tapered. These poor outcomes raise the question of whether the efficacy of opioid detoxifications can be improved by combining them with effective psychosocial interventions. That question was the rationale for the Bickel et al. (1997) study involving a comparison of the CRA plus vouchers treatment described above and a standard form of drug-abuse counseling commonly used with opioid-dependent clients (Ball & Ross, 1991). The subjects were 39 individuals undergoing a buprenorphine detoxification. Buprenorphine is a partial mu-opioid agonist that is currently being evaluated as a substitution pharmacotherapy for opioid dependence (Bickel & Amass, 1995). One notable change in the CRA plus vouchers treatment in this study was a modification in the voucher program so that one-half of the available vouchers could be earned via opioid-free urinalysis test results and the other half by participating in activities specified as part of CRA therapy.

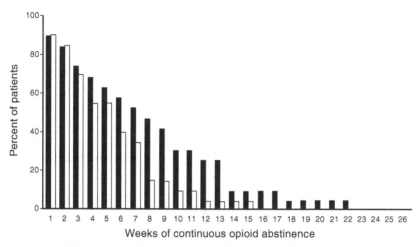

Figure 7.5 The height of each bar represents the percentage of subjects documented through urinalysis to have achieved a duration of continuous abstinence from illicit opioids equal to the number of weeks indicated. Note that the weeks of continuous abstinence could occur anywhere within the 26-week study. Filled bars represent the CRA plus vouchers group and unfilled bars the drug-abuse counseling group. Reprinted with permission from Bickel et al., 1997.

Subjects assigned to the CRA plus vouchers group were significantly more likely to complete the 24-week detoxification protocol (53% versus 20%) and achieved longer periods of documented opioid abstinence (Figure 7.5). There were no other significant differences between the two groups. This study demonstrates that the CRA plus vouchers treatment can be extended to the opioid-dependent population, and that outcomes in detoxification protocols can be enhanced by adding an effective psychosocial intervention.

Maintenance study

The maintenance study by Abbott et al. (1998*b*) involved methadone, which is a synthetic opioid agonist of the morphine type and the medication most commonly used in maintenance protocols (Ball & Ross, 1991). While maintenance protocols are efficacious when an adequate dose of medication is used, problems with ongoing drug abuse, unemployment and other psychosocial problems are common. Hence, there remains clinical and scientific interest in assessing how psychosocial interventions can improve the efficacy of opioid maintenance protocols.

One hundred and eighty-one patients were randomized to three groups and followed for 6 months after intake. The three groups were standard counseling ($n = 67$), CRA ($n = 52$), and CRA with relapse prevention ($n = 62$). The relapse prevention sessions were mostly delivered after the 6-month follow-up period, and thus the two CRA conditions were combined for analyses focused on outcomes during months 1–6. Of the 181 patients randomized, 165 were considered engaged in treatment (attended three or more treatment sessions) and contributed to assessments of outcome. Patients attended 20 treatment sessions in the standard and CRA groups. Patients in all groups received equivalent doses of methadone in the range of 60–70 mg daily. CRA was similar to that described above, but did not include a voucher component.

Significantly larger percentages of patients in the CRA groups (89%) than in the standard group (78%) achieved three consecutive weeks of opiate abstinence. Additionally, the CRA groups demonstrated significantly greater pre- to post-treatment improvements on the ASI drug composite scores than did the standard counseling group (Table 7.2). There were no significant retention differences between the treatment groups, which is to be expected in maintenance therapy with methadone doses in the 60- to 70-mg range.

Another critical outcome variable followed over time in this study was the reduction of risk-taking behavior, including injection drug use and high-risk sexual behavior. Overall risk behaviors decreased significantly although comparably in all treatment groups (Abbott et al., 1998a, b).

These results provided important new information supporting the efficacy of CRA in enhancing outcomes achieved with methadone-maintenance therapy. Moreover, this study provided the first demonstration of the efficacy of CRA with illicit-drug abusers when delivered apart from the voucher-based incentive program.

The study examining contingent vouchers used a within-subject reversal design to assess their efficacy in 13 methadone-maintenance patients (Silverman et al., 1996b). These patients consistently used illicit opioids during a 5-week period of baseline monitoring. Next, a 12-week voucher-based incentive program was introduced wherein patients earned vouchers contingent on opioid-negative urinalysis results following the same protocol as described above in the studies of cocaine-dependent individuals. The 12-week intervention period was followed by an 8-week return to baseline period. The percentage of urine specimens negative for opioids was significantly greater during the contingent incentive period than either of the baseline periods, demonstrating the efficacy of that incentive program for

Table 7.2. *Comparison of 151 patients receiving standard therapy (n = 55) or Community Reinforcement Therapy (n = 96) at intake and after 6 months*

Variable	Intake		6 months		Time effect[a]	Group effect[b]
	Standard	CRA	Standard	CRA		
ASI mean composite scores[c]						
Medical	0.17 (0.29)[d]	0.16 (0.29)	0.13 (0.27)	0.16 (0.29)	NS	NS
Employment	0.66 (0.30)	0.70 (0.30)	0.58 (0.32)	0.66 (0.32)	<0.01	NS
Alcohol	0.05 (0.09)	0.08 (0.17)	0.04 (0.11)	0.04 (0.13)	<0.05	NS
Drug	0.30 (0.12)	0.29 (0.11)	0.16 (0.11)	0.13 (0.09)	<0.001	0.044
Legal	0.17 (0.24)	0.14 (0.20)	0.07 (0.15)	0.06 (0.14)	<0.001	NS
Family/social	0.14 (0.19)	0.10 (0.18)	0.12 (0.18)	0.08 (0.17)	NS	NS
Psychological	0.13 (0.16)	0.17 (0.18)	0.08 (0.16)	0.08 (0.16)	<0.001	NS
Risk assessment battery	0.18 (0.12)	0.17 (0.12)	0.09 (0.08)	0.09 (0.09)	<0.001	NS
Social adjustment scales-SR	2.16 (0.50)	2.20 (0.63)	2.01(0.54)	1.96 (0.62)	<0.001	NS
Beck Depression Inventory	12.94 (10.06)	14.00 (9.73)	8.02 (8.07)	7.03 (7.88)	<0.001	NS
SCL-90	51.50 (46.76)	66.18 (52.86)	41.50 (52.22)	44.98 (48.45)	<0.01	NS

[a] Significance of F values for the time factor on 2 (group) × 2 (time) repeated-measure ANOVAs to determine improvement across conditions from intake to 6 months.

[b] Significance of F values for the one-way ANCOVA to determine group differences at 6 months using intake scores as covariate.

[c] Range is 0 to 1. Higher scores indicate greater problem severity. Composite scores reflect the 30 days prior to treatment and 6-month evaluation.

[d] Standard deviations in parentheses.

Reprinted with permission from Abbott et al., 1998b.

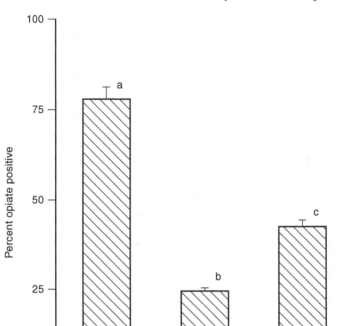

Figure 7.6 Mean percent of urinalysis test results positive for illicit-opioid use during baseline, voucher, and return-to-baseline conditions. Error bars represent ± SEM. Letters above the bars represent results from *post hoc* comparisons; bars that do not have a letter in common are significantly different from each other ($p \leqslant 0.01$). Reprinted with permission from Silverman et al., 1996*b*.

decreasing opioid abuse in these patients (Figure 7.6). While the second baseline period involved more opioid use than the intervention period, opiate use during the second baseline period remained significantly below levels observed in the initial baseline period, suggesting some continuing benefit from the contingent incentives.

Summary and conclusions

In this chapter we reviewed positive results from a series of well-controlled clinical trials supporting the efficacy of CRA treatments for cocaine and opioid dependence. The fact that much of the research on the use of CRA in the treatment of cocaine and opioid dependence has involved voucher-based incentives merits comment. The evidence is clear that vouchers are an effective element. Conceptually, the vouchers intervention is congruent with the operant conceptual framework of CRA and thus reasonably can be considered as simply an additional element of the CRA treatment package. It is worth remembering that monitored disulfiram therapy and several other elements of what is now considered the basic CRA treatment were not part of the original intervention. Rather, they were added later as improvements of CRA (Azrin, 1976). Perhaps the vouchers should be thought of similarly. However the vouchers are considered, CRA has made contributions to the treatment of cocaine and opioid dependence apart from them. The idea of using disulfiram therapy with individuals abusing alcohol and cocaine, for example, arose directly out of the use of CRA with that population (*see* Higgins et al., 1993*a*), and has now been demonstrated to be efficacious independently of the other CRA elements (Carroll et al., 1998). Comparisons of the results of CRA without vouchers to standard drug-abuse counseling suggest greater efficacy for CRA. More substantially, the trial by Abbott and colleagues (Abbott et al., 1998*b*) with opioid-dependent individuals did not involve vouchers and yet the CRA treatment resulted in greater reductions in opioid use than standard drug-abuse counseling. Delivered with or without vouchers, CRA represents an efficacious treatment that can enhance treatment outcomes with cocaine- and opioid-dependent patients.

A theoretical note worth underscoring is that the research reviewed in this chapter illustrates the fundamental importance of the principle of reinforcement to understanding and effectively treating cocaine, opioid and other drug dependence. An extensive basic-science literature demonstrates the role of pharmacologically based reinforcement in the genesis and maintenance of drug use and abuse (Griffiths, Bigelow & Henningfield, 1980). In addition to pharmacological reinforcement, there is sound scientific evidence demonstrating the contribution of socially mediated reinforcement to the development and maintenance of drug use and abuse (Griffiths, Bigelow & Liebson, 1978). The research reviewed herein on CRA demonstrates how that same reinforcement principle can be systematically applied in the effective treatment of cocaine and opioid dependence. Recognizing the importance of reinforcement to substance dependence and integrating systematic use of that principle into clinical efforts to reduce cocaine and opioid dependence has the potential to substantially improve treatment outcomes.

Treatments based on well established scientific concepts and principles can generally be well specified. That holds true for CRA. Clinician manuals were used in each of the studies described in this chapter, and, as is noted above, two of the CRA treatment manuals have been published (Budney & Higgins, 1998; Meyers & Smith, 1995). Well specified procedures permit the type of successful replication and extensions of CRA that are described in this volume. They should also help to facilitate the important next step of successfully disseminating these treatments to community substance-abuse clinics and other agencies involved in the effort to reduce cocaine and opioid dependence.

8

Community Reinforcement and Family Training (CRAFT)

ROBERT J. MEYERS, WILLIAM R. MILLER AND JANE ELLEN SMITH

Background and research

It has become clearly evident that the behavior of an individual with a substance-abuse problem can have a pronounced negative impact on the lives of family members and friends (Collins, Leonard & Searles, 1990; Orford & Harwin, 1982; Velleman et al., 1993). Paolino and McCrady (1977) estimated that for every excessive drinker there are five others who suffer directly. Problems experienced by these significant others range from mild verbal abuse to severe physical violence. Other negative effects documented by the loved ones of substance-abusing individuals include depressed mood, physical complaints, low self-confidence, and high levels of anxiety (Brown et al., 1995; Kogan & Jacobson, 1965; Moos, Finney & Gamble, 1982). Additionally, these concerned significant others (CSOs) report elevated levels of marital distress (Thomas & Ager, 1993).

A scientifically based model designed to help these CSOs engage resistant substance abusers into treatment was not available until the early 1980s. Traditionally, assistance for family members was limited to an Al-Anon-based approach and the Johnson Institute intervention. The former taught individuals to detach from substance abusers, and the latter utilized a surprise group confrontation. Importantly, the behavioral program called the Community Reinforcement Approach (CRA; Azrin et al., 1982; Hunt & Azrin, 1973) has always operated with quite a different view of the role that a CSO could play in the treatment of substance abuse. For example, CRA has enlisted CSOs successfully as disulfiram monitors, partners in marital counseling, active agents in resocialization and reinforcement programs, and detection monitors for relapse (Azrin, 1976; Azrin et al., 1982; Hunt & Azrin, 1973; Smith, Meyers & Delaney, 1998). The related CRAFT program (Community Reinforcement and Family Training) was developed with the belief that since family members can

147

make important contributions in other areas of treatment, they can play a powerful role in helping to engage a resistant loved one into therapy. Most CSOs can also benefit from counseling that teaches them to become more independent and to take better care of themselves.

CRAFT uses an overall positive approach and steers clear of confrontation. The program is similar to CRA in that it emphasizes learning new skills to cope with old problems. In fact, many of the actual skills training strategies used in CRA are also used in CRAFT (*see* Meyers & Smith, 1995). Some of CRAFT's basic components include discussing personal safety issues, outlining the context in which substance-abusing behaviors occur, teaching CSOs how to utilize positive reinforcers for both the substance user and themselves, and emphasizing lifestyle changes for the CSO.

Sisson and Azrin (1986) conducted the first randomized study examining the viability of using community-based reinforcement procedures with a problem drinker's CSO. They randomly assigned 12 CSOs to receive either an early version of CRAFT (Community Reinforcement Training: CRT) or a disease model/Al-Anon approach. In the CRT condition, six of seven resistant alcoholics entered treatment after a mean of 58.2 days and an average of 7.2 CSO sessions. Interestingly, the drinkers had already reduced their mean consumption by more than half by the time they started the program. In contrast, none of the traditional group's drinkers sought treatment.

In a recent trial funded by the National Institute on Alcohol Abuse and Alcoholism (NIAAA), 130 CSOs were randomized into one of three different engagement approaches: (1) Al-Anon facilitation therapy, which was designed to encourage involvement in the 12-step program and to get resistant drinkers to enter formal treatment; (2) a Johnson Institute intervention, which prepared the CSO for a confrontational family meeting that led to formal treatment; and (3) the CRAFT approach, which taught behavioral change skills and new strategies for guiding the drinker into treatment. All three therapies were manual based and consisted of 12 hours of planned contact. Assessment interviews were conducted by individuals who were uninformed regarding group assignment.

In terms of the results, the CRAFT approach was significantly more effective in engaging resistant problem drinkers into treatment (64%) as compared with the more commonly used Al-Anon (13%) and Johnson Institute (30%) interventions (Miller, Meyers & Tonigan, 1999). As far as session attendance, the CSOs in the Al-Anon group participated in slightly more of the 12 scheduled sessions (95%) than did the CSOs in the CRAFT group (89%), while CSOs assigned to the Johnson Institute intervention attended only 53% of the sessions. Nevertheless, one should note that the high attendance rates for the Al-Anon group did not serve as an advantage in terms of engaging their loved ones into treatment. If one specifically examines the length of time required by the CRAFT-trained CSOs to get their resistant drinker into treatment, the median number of days was 47, with an average of 4.7 CSO sessions being completed. In terms of CSOs' functioning, although we found no between-group differences, there were marked improvements over time on all five dependent measures for the CSO. These were in the areas of depression (Beck Depression Inventory: Beck et al., 1961), anger (State-Trait Anger Expression Inventory: Forgays et al., 1998; Spielberger, 1996), family cohesion and conflict (Family Environment Scale: Moos & Moos, 1986) and general happiness (Happiness Scale: Azrin et al., 1973).

A modified and updated CRAFT approach was designed to engage illicit-drug-using adults into treatment (Meyers & Smith, 1997; Meyers, Dominguez & Smith, 1996). In this noncontrolled National Institute on Drug Abuse (NIDA) demonstration trial, CSO therapy attendance was excellent. The 62 participants attended 87% of their 12 offered sessions. During the 6-month study period, 46 of the 62 CSOs (74%) succeeded in engaging their resistant loved one into treatment. The average length of CSO treatment before engagement was 4.8 sessions, or 45 days from the first counseling appointment. Reported abstinence both from illicit drugs and alcohol increased significantly for drug users engaged in treatment, but not for the unengaged cases (Meyers et al., 1999). In addition, all CSOs showed significant reductions from baseline in depression, anger, anxiety, and negative physical symptoms.

Overall, our findings support with reasonable confidence the belief that CRAFT is a substantially more effective program than the commonly utilized approaches for engaging unmotivated substance abusers. Furthermore, the CRAFT studies indicate that successful intervention is possible not only through spouses, but through other family members as well. In fact, we observed in both trials a significantly greater advantage for parents (relative to partners) in engaging resistant substance abusers. Our findings clearly show that CSOs need not wait for substance abusers to find their own intrinsic motivation for change. Future research may demonstrate that these methods are applicable to the engagement of treatment-resistant individuals with other life problems as well.

CRAFT procedures

With a behavioral philosophy similar to the "parent" CRA program, CRAFT is a comprehensive set of procedures designed to help CSOs reduce their emotional suffering, engage their resistant loved ones into treatment, and increase happiness between CSOs and their problem users (Meyers & Smith, 1997; Meyers & Wolfe, 1998; Meyers, Dominguez & Smith, 1996; Meyers, Smith & Miller, 1998; Smith, Meyers & Waldorf, 1999). The intent is to empower CSOs to take control where feasible, but never at the expense of taking care of themselves. CRAFT relies upon skills training and other strategies that lead to personal independence and improved self-efficacy and self-esteem. CRAFT procedures primarily focus on:

1. Developing a trusting therapeutic relationship.
2. Preparing the CSO to recognize and safely respond to any potential for domestic violence, particularly when the behavioral changes are being introduced at home.
3. Completing two functional analyses; the first to identify the substance user's triggers for using alcohol or drugs and the consequences, and the second to profile the user's triggers for nonusing, pro-social behavior and its consequences.
4. Working to improve communication with the substance user.
5. Showing the CSO how to effectively use positive reinforcement and negative consequences such that they discourage a loved one's harmful using behavior.
6. Teaching the CSO methods for decreasing stress in general, and emphasizing the importance of having sufficient "rewards" in his or her own life.
7. Instructing the CSO in the most effective ways to suggest treatment to the substance user, and helping to identify the most appropriate times.
8. Laying the groundwork for having treatment available immediately for the user in the event that the decision is made to begin therapy, and discussing the need for the CSO to support the drinker or drug user during treatment.

The CRAFT program must be delivered by a therapist who is not only well versed in the procedures, but who also has sound fundamental counseling skills, such as supportiveness, empathy, and a genuine caring attitude. In addition, a CRAFT therapist is energetic, directive, and engaging. This enthusiasm helps motivate the client to make difficult changes. Also, the style lends itself to having the client open up sufficiently such that a rich supply of potential reinforcers is revealed.

Building rapport and trust

A CSO will be more receptive to trying new behaviors if there is trust in the therapist and the therapy system, so we take the necessary time to build rapport and gain trust before any new procedures are introduced and negotiated. This is critical, since the CSO may feel confused, humiliated, disgraced, shameful, guilty, or even responsible with regard to the loved one's unhealthy behavior. Initially we simply listen carefully and reassure the CSO that these feelings are natural and expected. One way we normalize the CSO's story is to discuss similar cases, emphasizing how people react in the best way they can at the time. We then find a specific problem area and briefly review alternative ways to approach it, while mentioning that others have learned to address comparable issues with training and support.

Another technique for building rapport with the client is to give a brief overview of the goals and philosophy of CRAFT. This is also a good time to answer any questions, which in turn may help the client to gain ownership of the program and reduce anxiety. Additionally, this affords us a suitable time to use positive reinforcement in the form of praise for all the effort the CSO already has dedicated to the relationship. Throughout this process we strive to demonstrate knowledge and competence, so the client begins to believe that solutions can be found. Eventually trust replaces skepticism, and the process moves forward.

During this early stage of treatment we must also identify the "reinforcers" that a CSO will receive for taking new steps. In other words, these reinforcers are the prizes the CSO is willing to work hard for in therapy. Examples might include: improvement in family finances, greater marital satisfaction, better sexual gratification, enhanced relationships with children and other family members, and greater enjoyment of social and recreational activities. Whenever possible, we discuss potential benefits that are specific to the CSO. The following dialogue gives an example of how to use the client's reinforcers to encourage her to try something new:

THERAPIST I understand how difficult it is for you to discuss these issues with your husband, but I think it's necessary.

CLIENT I just don't know if I can ask him for more money. He thinks what he gives me is enough to run the house and take care of the kids.

THERAPIST I know this is difficult, but I'm going to help. We can practise what to say, and even when to say it. Remember, you did say earlier that one of your goals was to have your husband get more involved with the kids. Maybe this is one way you can get him involved.

CLIENT I'm not sure what you mean. I just know how upset he gets when we talk about money. That's why I usually just make do with what I have.

THERAPIST That's one way to deal with the problem. But how about if we approach it from a different angle? What would he say if you asked him his opinion on what sort of school clothes and supplies to buy your kids? If we can get him engaged in the conversation, then you could tactfully bring up the money issue; at least as it pertains to school items. Let's role-play this situation. You take the role of your husband and I'm going to start our planned conversation acting like I'm you.

This example shows how important it is to know what motivates clients, for this information can be used to support them to make necessary changes. In addition to encouraging the CSO to try new strategies, these reinforcers can be used later to provide a frustrated CSO with a rationale for remaining in treatment. For example, assume a CSO states that the most important thing for her is to raise the children in a caring home environment, and yet she is only willing to half-heartedly attempt a few of CRAFT's behavioral procedures with her alcohol-dependent husband. Not surprisingly, nothing changes and she feels defeated. We can then remind her about her reinforcer, namely having a caring environment for her children, in order to motivate the CSO to actively work towards obtaining it. And frequently the first step is getting the husband into treatment.

Domestic violence precautions

It is important to proceed carefully when supporting a CSO's efforts to introduce behavioral changes with a substance user, given the significant association between substance abuse and domestic violence (Coleman & Straus, 1986; Gondolf & Foster, 1991; Leonard & Jacob, 1988; Stith, Crossman & Bischof, 1991). CRAFT's initial procedures include an assessment of the potential for violence, usually with an instrument such as the Conflict Tactics Scale (Straus, 1979). If a history of violence is discovered, it is useful to conduct a functional analysis of the behaviors that typically precede and follow the violence. For example, assume a CSO describes the following situation:

Some days when my husband comes home from work he appears nervous and starts to pace around the house. When I ask him what's wrong, he tells me to stop bugging him and to just leave him alone. If I leave him alone for a little while and then go back to see how he's doing, he typically gets agitated and his voice grows loud. If he heads for the basement, I know I'm in trouble. I know that's where he hides liquor. Once he goes to the basement I know he's going to start to drink. When he starts up the stairs from the basement I listen carefully, because if his footsteps are heavy and slow I know he's going to be violent. I hate hearing the sound of his heavy footsteps on the basement stairs.

The advanced recognition of escalating danger can become routine with proper awareness training. The CSO first learns the precursors of her husband's violent behavior (appearing nervous and pacing, yelling at her to leave him alone, becoming agitated and loud, going downstairs to the basement, making heavy and slow footsteps on the staircase). These "signs" become her signal to respond in a different manner. The new responses are designed to prevent or curtail the violent behavior. An example of a new safer response would be leaving him alone indefinitely when he appears nervous and agitated, and simply stating that she is in the other room if and when he wants to talk. CRAFT devotes time to role-playing these new reactions that have the potential for decreasing violent behavior.

Since altering the CSO's normal behavior in any way could elicit a further negative reaction from the substance abuser, a back-up safety plan is prepared in the event that violence threatens. CRAFT teaches CSOs who have reported violent episodes how to take specific steps to stay safe. One option is to learn about domestic violence centers and the use of a safe house. Or the CSO may choose to retreat to the home of a friend or relative instead. Regardless, CSOs are taught to have a bag packed with proper clothing, credentials, money and other necessary articles in the event that they leave the house suddenly for a few days.

Functional analyses

From the onset, the CSO is invited to try new strategies that may be instrumental in changing the drinking or using behavior, and in getting the individual to seek treatment. With regard to the former, one new procedure for most CSOs is the functional analysis. As noted in Chapter 3, CRA utilizes two different kinds of functional analyses: one for substance-abusing behavior and one for nonusing, pleasurable activities. The CRAFT program similarly uses both types of functional analyses, but this time the CSO completes these forms for the substance abuser.

When the CSO is first asked to outline the loved one's pattern of substance use, the emphasis is on the triggers for the using behavior. It is important for the CSO to be cognizant of the user's antecedents to alcohol or drug use, so that strategies can be taught to alter the CSO's behavior at these times. For example, assume the wife of a drinker realizes in the course of doing a functional analysis that a trigger for her husband is anger towards his boss. Whenever he arrives home and slams his car keys on the counter while muttering about needing to find another job, she now knows that his next move will be to head back out to the liquor store. In hearing this scenario, we explore the wife's options for helping her husband respond to his anger in some healthier manner, such as by suggesting that they immediately take a walk together or go to a movie.

We next review the consequences so the CSO can recall vividly how he or she is affected by and reacts to the loved one's using behavior. In particular, the CSO's responses to the drinking or using behavior are highlighted in the event that these reactions are inadvertently helping to maintain the substance-abusing behavior. In such cases, more adaptive coping responses eventually are taught. The functional analysis is sometimes supplemented with an instrument specifically designed to identify spouses' ineffectual coping strategies, such as the Spouse Enabling Inventory or the Spouse Sobriety Influence Inventory (Thomas, Yoshioka & Ager, 1996).

A second, separate functional analysis is then completed so that the CSO can identify antecedents for several of the loved one's pleasurable, nonsubstance-abusing behaviors. This forms the basis for later interventions that will attempt to increase the frequency of enjoyable nonusing activities. The CSO has a wealth of knowledge about the functioning and habits of the substance user, yet knowing how and when to utilize this information is the key to positive behavior change. We assist the CSO in exploring activities that elicit pro-social behaviors from the loved one. Then the extent to which the substance abuser actually enjoys these activities is determined, since without considerable reinforcement value they will never be able to compete with the abusive behavior. Next the CSO generates a list of possible reinforcers that can be used to reward nonusing behavior (*see* "Use of positive reinforcement" section for a full explanation).

Communication training

CRAFT is for family members and friends who hope to maintain their relationship with the resistant substance user, but who want it to change in a positive direction. Typically it is useful to start by examining the manner in which the CSO currently communicates with the loved one. It is not uncommon to see fairly negative interchanges at this crisis point in the relationship. But if the communication pattern continues to be dominated by reciprocal blaming and defensiveness, the CSO will have minimal success in positively influencing the loved one's using behavior and eventually engaging him or her into treatment. So the CSO is taught how to communicate in a way that will maximize the chances of the problem user listening and responding in kind. CRAFT relies upon the positive communication skills training outlined in the CRA program (See Chapter 3 this volume, or Meyers & Smith, 1995, pp. 163–70).

Use of positive reinforcement

The CSO is in a unique position to support or discourage the loved one's substance use even through modest changes in the CSO's own behavior. Unfortunately, most CSOs' customary attempts at managing the behavior tend to be ineffective and unsystematic. Some examples include constantly nagging the user to stop, emotional pleading, discarding the substance abuser's alcohol or illicit drugs, getting intoxicated to "show them what it's like", or even threatening the user. Typically we discuss the limitations of these old, ineffective approaches. We then present the notion of teaching the CSO to systematically arrange positive consequences for *non*using behaviors, so the substance abuser's behavior is altered in a favorable direction.

We begin by again explaining the concept of a positive reinforcer, or a reward, to the CSO. The CSO is then asked to identify several small reinforcers that could be introduced when the loved one is *not* using, such as preparing the individual's favorite meal, discussing the user's favorite topic, offering verbal praise or support for sobriety, suggesting a romantic encounter, or just spending time with the individual. Regardless of the reinforcer selected, it is necessary to explore whether it is powerful enough to compete with the substance-abusing behavior. We next explain the critical importance of introducing the rewards at a time when the user is clean, sober and not hungover. The CSO is queried about being able to recognize when the loved one is under the influence of even a small amount of alcohol or drugs (see Meyers, Dominguez & Smith, 1996, p. 277). Finally, we train the CSO to verbally link the reward with nonusing behavior. For example, the CSO might practise saying, "You know, sometimes I absolutely adore you and cherish our time together. I just can't get enough of you. And it finally dawned on me that this is the time we spend together when you're straight. So that's when I want to spend my time with you. If you begin using, I'll have to excuse myself and leave. I thought it was important for you to know how I really feel."

Sometimes the anger that has built up over time in a CSO toward the substance user temporarily blocks the CSO's willingness to use positive reinforcement. Other CSOs point out that it would not be appropriate to do anything special for the user, since this could be considered "enabling" or rescuing behavior. We quickly clarify that positive reinforcement is not an enabling behavior when it is introduced only when the user is *clean and sober*. We sometimes encourage tentative changes in the CSO's behavior through the sampling procedure introduced in the CRA model. In this application the technique teaches a CSO to "sample" a new behavior for a limited period of time in order to give the process a chance to work (Azrin et al., 1982; Meyers & Smith, 1995; Miller & Page, 1991; Smith & Meyers, 1995). So a reluctant CSO is asked to simply experiment with introducing positive reinforcement at nonusing times, and to observe whether it creates any movement toward the ultimate goal of reducing the user's alcohol or drug use.

A checklist of the skills required before implementing the use of positive reinforcement with the substance user follows:

1. The CSO can describe the concept and has identified appropriate positive reinforcers.
2. The CSO has the capability of delivering suitable reinforcers, as demonstrated in role-plays and possibly by practising first with another family member or friend.
3. The CSO has discussed possible resentment for being expected to give rewards to someone who has caused so much pain.
4. The CSO understands that the reward should only be introduced when the user is clean, sober and not hungover.

5. The CSO is aware of a variety of possible consequences of this new behavior, and is prepared to address any problematic negative reactions.

One way to teach the CSO about positive reinforcement is to model the behavior during the treatment sessions. Not only does this provide a real-life example, but the CSO can experience first hand how it feels to get positive feedback for specific behavior.

Use of negative consequences

In addition to being taught how to link positive rewards to nondrinking/nonusing behavior, the CSO learns how *not* to reward unwanted behaviors. In order to do this we begin by discussing ways in which the client may be inadvertently supporting the substance-abusing behavior. An example of this is the CSO who calls in sick for the drinker whenever he has a hangover. Once the CSO has generated examples of similar types of unwanted behaviors and their consequences, we move into a solution-focused mode. This entails having the CSO pick one of the loved one's problematic behaviors that the CSO is willing to work on. Failed previous attempts to prevent the behavior are reviewed, and a short functional analysis of the behavior is completed. In particular, the negative consequences created by the behavior for both the user and the CSO are highlighted.

When it comes time to settle on an intervention, we always first explore the feasibility of using positive reinforcement to change unwanted behaviors. But since frequently this needs to be supplemented by the use of negative consequences as well, these are discussed at length. Typically the negative consequences are simply the natural consequences for the substance-abusing behavior. For example, if the drinker sleeps in late and misses their bus to get to work, normally they would suffer the wrath of their boss. But if the CSO wakes them and makes sure they catch the bus, perhaps even drives them, they have escaped those negative consequences. Importantly, we never suggest behavior changes for the CSO without first considering the potential reactions of the substance abuser. Then role-plays are conducted so that the CSO can practise introducing each new behavior. As part of the role-plays, we illustrate possible negative responses by the substance abuser, since the CSO must be comfortable handling a variety of scenarios before trying a new behavior. One reasonable plan in anticipation of a strong negative reaction from the user is for the CSO to be ready to leave the house. Presenting the substance-abusing individual with a "time out" sends a clear message that abuse in any form will not be tolerated.

In conclusion, when any modification of a CSO's approach to substance-using behavior is being taught, it is always preferable to support the use of positive reinforcement if possible. However, in some cases the repeated attempts to positively reinforce the drinker's nonusing behavior fail, and consequently the introduction of negative consequences may be warranted. We have found that CRAFT therapists commonly encourage CSOs to use a combination of both positive reinforcement and negative, natural consequences.

Teaching CSOs how to reward themselves

Another goal of CRAFT is to help the CSO improve the quality of his or her own life, regardless of whether the user enters treatment. So CRAFT encourages the CSO to make positive lifestyle changes independent of the loved one. As a step towards doing this, the CSO often completes a functional analysis for his or her own pro-social behaviors. Once the triggers are outlined and the consequences are reviewed, plans are made to increase the frequency of these activities. Interestingly, we spend considerable time and energy discussing this entire issue, since CSOs often feel guilty about engaging in pleasurable activities on their own. At the same time, if the CSOs can master identifying and engaging in enjoyable activities for themselves, it may be easier for them to learn to set up pleasurable, competing behaviors for the substance abuser.

Getting the substance user into treatment

Research has demonstrated the difficulty in engaging and retaining an individual with substance-abuse problems in treatment (Baekeland & Lundwall, 1975; Ellis et al., 1992; Stark & Campbell, 1988). According to Foote and colleagues (1994), "The issues of engagement and retention must assume prominence in the development of new treatment approaches." As noted already, several clinical trials have shown CRAFT to be significantly more effective at engaging resistant individuals than the commonly used methods (Meyers et al., 1999; Miller, Meyers & Tonigan, 1999; Sisson & Azrin, 1986). Furthermore, CRAFT is successful not only in working with spouses, but with other family members of problem drinkers and drug users as well. Parents were quite successful in engaging their adult children, but grandfathers and grandmothers were at least as effective.

Every CSO has a unique set of problems, yet there are common techniques that can be used to engage most substance abusers. If probing determines that violence is not an issue, we can proceed right into an engagement mode. As part of doing this we sometimes hear CSOs say that they have given up; that they no longer discuss with their loved one the using behavior. So before we can move on to specific strategies it must be established that the CSO is willing to try one last attempt at helping this loved one refrain from using drugs or alcohol.

Typical questions used to begin the engagement training process are, "What have you done in the past that has been successful in getting your loved one to reduce his/her use?" and "What have you done in the past that has *not* worked?" Then we ask, "What do you think your loved one would say right now if you invited him/her to come to treatment?" With a careful discussion and analysis of these behaviors we begin to get a picture of how to approach this particular individual.

At this stage in the CSO's treatment we repeatedly ask ourselves the question, "What would get this resistant substance abuser to simply 'sample' treatment?" After much preparation and practice the CSO tries several different ways to encourage the loved one to accompany the CSO to therapy. One approach that sometimes works is inviting users to come in to help the CSO. Since in most cases the substance abuse has caused a variety of problems between the CSO and the user, it does not appear odd when the CSO asks the individual to enter couples treatment to help with a problem that is not specifically related to substance abuse. Other problem areas may appear less threatening, thus making it more likely that the drinker will escort the CSO to at least one therapy session. The responsibility then lies with us. Once rapport is built and the user is part of therapy, over time the process will inevitably begin to focus on substance abuse. The CSO is told in advance that all roads lead back to the cause of the problems, substance abuse, and that if the process unfolds naturally, user compliance in therapy is much higher.

Timing is everything! Knowing precisely when to invite the substance user into treatment has a lot to do with the comfort level of the CSO as well as with the hypothesized reaction of the substance abuser. If a CSO has told the loved one about being in therapy, the user sometimes asks curiously about what is going on in the CSO's program. It is also common for the user to ask the CSO why he or she has been acting strangely. These tend to be ideal times for the CSO to bring up the topic of treatment. The CSO may choose to only hint to the user about the purpose of treatment, or may clearly spell out the specific intent of the CRAFT program. Regardless, an invitation to attend a session typically follows.

Rapid intake procedure

It is critical to lay the groundwork for a rapid intake of the substance user once the decision to enter treatment is made. The chances of treatment beginning at all drop markedly if an ambivalent user is placed on a waiting list. Once the individual enters treatment, CRA is recommended (Azrin, 1976; Azrin et al., 1982; Hunt & Azrin, 1973; Meyers & Smith, 1995).

Getting the loved one to enter treatment is really only the start. We always discuss the importance of the CSO staying active in the user's therapy. The structure of therapy changes, however, because now the CSO and the substance user present as a couple in need of help. We also prepare the CSO for the possibility that the user will enter treatment only to drop out prematurely. Again the CSO is reminded that CRAFT is an ongoing process. When a user leaves treatment early, it is just one step in the program, and more work needs to be done to encourage the individual to return.

Conclusion

Research over the years has repeatedly demonstrated the considerable difficulty in engaging and retaining an individual in treatment with sub-stance-abuse problems (Baekeland & Lundwall, 1975; Ellis et al., 1992; Stark & Campbell, 1988). Two CRAFT projects, one sponsored by NIAAA and a second by NIDA, have shown that engagement is not only possible, but probable. Through these trials it has also become apparent that CRAFT is substantially more effective in engaging unmotivated substance abusers in treatment than are the two approaches most commonly used for this purpose in the U.S. And research questions are still being addressed, as there are two NIDA-funded CRAFT trials currently underway. Additionally, a treatment development study is being conducted to explore the effectiveness of CRAFT with substance-abusing adolescents and their families.

9

Summary and Reflections

WILLIAM R. MILLER AND ROBERT J. MEYERS

The chapters of this book have told the story of the Community Reinforcement Approach (CRA) from its very beginning in the late 1960s through current research at the start of a new century. The studies described here have involved nearly a thousand clients treated with CRA for alcohol and illicit drug problems. Most of these clients have had relatively severe substance dependence, and many (as exemplified in the study with homeless adults in Chapter 6) have had many other serious life problems and diagnoses as well. There is no sense in which any of these were particularly "good prognosis" populations.

But then prognosis, like motivation, is not merely a matter of client characteristics. Prognosis occurs in the context of available treatments. Many diseases that at one time were typically terminal are now readily treatable. Similarly, there are now effective and even brief treatments for psychological problems that just a few decades ago were thought to be relatively intractable. Prognosis also has to do with the availability of effective treatment methods. It was the promise of effectiveness that drew us to CRA. The Azrin studies, outlined in Chapter 2, provided some of the strongest empirical evidence for the efficacy of any treatment method for alcohol dependence. Yet in spite of promising evidence, CRA was rarely used, and most practitioners had never even heard of it. We wanted to see whether CRA would work in our hands, in a very different culture from rural Illinois where it was born, and with some of the "toughest" clients we could find, in a real-life treatment agency.

Our collaboration is now entering its third decade, and we know much more than when we began. We are also much better clinical researchers than when we started. Treatment outcome research is no simple task, and is certainly not for those who like immediate results. Yet in another sense we have enjoyed relatively rapid reinforcement hundreds of times during the course of these studies, in the positive outcomes of our individual clients.

Lessons learned

So what have we learned? Here is a concise summary of the results of more than a dozen trials spanning three decades, involving hundreds of clients and dozens of therapists, supported primarily by the National Institute on Alcohol Abuse and Alcoholism (NIAAA) and the National Institute on Drug Abuse (NIDA).

1. CRA works

This can't be said of many treatment methods with such confidence. In terms of experimental methodology, all of the tests of CRA's efficacy have been relatively stringent. CRA-based treatments have been tested, not against untreated or waiting list control groups, but in comparison with the most common, state-of-practice treatments available. In each and every one of these studies, in order to yield a positive outcome, CRA had to perform better than or add to the effectiveness of standard treatment methods already in common use. In each and every study it has done so. Through the original Azrin studies in Illinois, our first alcohol trial in New Mexico (Chapters 3–4), the Higgins studies with cocaine-dependent people in Vermont, the Abbott study with clients in methadone maintenance (Chapter 7), and the Sisson and Azrin (1986) and our own studies of unilateral CRAFT intervention (Chapter 8), the CRA-based treatment has yielded significantly better outcomes.

2. CRA is teachable

This is a technology that can be transferred. The procedures are well specified, and the approach is systematic and theory based. Dozens of therapists have delivered CRA in these trials over the years. Many of them were relative novices, graduate students at the beginning of their careers, and yet the outcomes have been excellent. It is also noteworthy that in a field where therapist differences seem to be the norm (e.g., Najavits & Weiss, 1994; Project MATCH Research Group, 1998), we have never found significant differences in the effectiveness of therapists delivering CRA, despite a wide range in their initial level of clinical experience.

Therapist differences probably do occur in the application of CRA, but clearly this is not a treatment approach that depends on charisma or a high degree of clinical experience and acumen. It can be learned and applied with reasonably consistent results.

3. Relapse prevention

We are not particularly fond of the popular concept of "relapse" (Miller, 1996), but relapse prevention is often stated as a goal of treatment. It appears to us that this is a reasonable description of the actual effects of CRA. Across studies, there is a pattern of initial suppression of substance use in CRA and also in other treatments with which it is compared. Across months of follow-up, however, outcomes remain relatively flat in CRA groups, whereas in comparison (standard treatment) conditions there tends to be more of a rebound toward original levels of use. To be sure, CRA is not the only treatment method with which this pattern has been observed (e.g., Project MATCH Research Group, 1997). The observed differences between CRA and traditional treatments, however, often appear in the maintenance of initial treatment gains. In some cases, these differences wash out over longer periods of follow-up (e.g., Chapter 4); in others, they remain (e.g., Chapter 6).

4. Involvement of significant others makes a difference

From its inception, CRA has focused on sources of reinforcement in the client's natural environment, and that usually means involving significant others. In one early study (Azrin et al., 1982), simply adding the disulfiram-compliance procedure to traditional treatment was enough for clients who were married, whereas for those who were single it took the full CRA to suppress drinking. In the first New Mexico study (Chapter 4), teaching a significant other the disulfiram-compliance procedure again improved the outcome of traditional treatment. In our CRAFT studies (Chapter 8), the drinking or drug use of the identified patient (IP) decreased during the course of unilateral intervention via the significant other, whether or not the IP ultimately entered treatment. Although we have not yet tested, by experimental design, whether involving a significant other improves outcomes from CRA treatment, these findings are consistent with the CRA view that it is possible to diminish substance use by altering reinforcement contingencies in the home environment.

5. Positive reinforcement works

This is no news to psychologists, but another general pattern in CRA research is that positive reinforcement can alter substance use. CRA has always emphasized the importance of using positive reinforcement throughout the therapy process. Beyond a large amount of experimental literature on the subject, the work of Higgins and his colleagues (Chapter 7) clearly shows that even contrived reinforcers (such as monetary vouchers) for abstinence can suppress drug use (Higgins & Silverman, 1999). Similarly, when family members are taught to alter their patterns of positive reinforcement, the IP's substance use declines. Other evidence indicates that positive reinforcement is more effective than negative reinforcement (withdrawing desired conditions) in altering substance use (e.g., Stitzer et al., 1986).

6. Broad spectrum response

We have found no client pretreatment characteristics that are consistent predictors of response to CRA. We have observed good results in the presence of high severity of dependence, multiple diagnoses, and homelessness. Indeed, Project MATCH (1997) provided little evidence that client attributes are robust predictors of differential response to cognitive-behavioral versus other approaches. CRA does not seem to be a treatment that should be reserved for certain kinds of clients, or should be shied away from when problems are more severe. As with other treatments, employment and social support for sobriety are associated with better overall outcomes (Project MATCH, 1997). In CRA, there are specific treatment procedures targeting these protective factors. CRA also seems to be applicable across cultural differences, having been applied with affluent and poor, rural and urban, and minority populations including Hispanics and African-Americans. The Na'nazhoozhi center in Gallup, New Mexico has offered a CRA-based treatment for alcohol and other drug problems among traditional Diné (Navajo) people (Miller, Meyers & Hiller-Sturmhöfel, 1999).

7. CRA need not be expensive

Based on the intensity of treatment described in the original CRA reports (Azrin, 1976; Hunt & Azrin, 1973), some have concluded that, while it is effective, CRA is not a method that can be provided within the cost constraints of real-life treatment systems. This is simply not so. Although there have certainly been expensive applications of CRA (Higgins et al., 1993*a*, *b*), significantly better outcomes (relative to traditional approaches) have been found with CRA-based treatments of five to eight sessions across a wide range of studies described in this volume. This amount of treatment is well within the normal bounds of managed care. CRA has also been adapted well in group therapy format (Smith, Meyers & Delaney, 1998). Some of the more staff-intensive components of CRA (such as a Job Club or social club) have been utilized by relatively few clients in some studies, and it is possible to offer effective CRA without these more costly components.

8. Disulfiram is not necessary

An unanswered question was the extent to which disulfiram, added by Azrin in 1976, is necessary to the efficacy of CRA. We can now answer confidently in the negative. This was a key experimental question in two of our trials (Chapters 4 and 6), and in neither case did the addition of disulfiram (with compliance training) improve the average efficacy of CRA. Interestingly, in two studies the addition of the CRA disulfiram-compliance procedure did improve the efficacy of traditional treatment (Azrin et al., 1982; Chapter 4).

Why hasn't CRA been used more broadly?

Despite evidence of efficacy in a long series of clinical trials, and the successful demonstration of the application of CRA in a broad range of nations and cultures, the fact remains that relatively few treatment programs use this approach. Why is that? It is a question we have asked ourselves often. Here are some of our thoughts.

Limited accessibility

George Hunt, Azrin's student and a driving force behind CRA, died tragically in a boating accident in the 1970s. Of others involved in the original Illinois studies, only two (Nathan Azrin and Robert Meyers) have continued to be actively involved in substance-abuse treatment. There have been no training programs in CRA. Stated simply, there have been too few experienced senior clinicians to promote and teach this approach. For two decades, CRA was accessible only through scientific journals, and reasonably obscure ones at that, with very limited "how to" descriptions of the approach. Until very recently, there were no manuals to guide therapists in the application of CRA (Meyers & Smith, 1995). This manual outlines the goals and procedures of each particular technique and provides a step-by-step guideline. At the time of writing, there are still no training videotapes.

The disease model

It has become almost fashionable to blame the disease model for all manner of systemic problems, a critical tradition that began with Jellinek (1960). Yet there is a sense in which this may be one important aspect of why CRA has not been more widely used, at least within the U.S. Whatever the specific mechanisms being emphasized, American-style disease models have looked almost exclusively within the individual for the cause of alcoholism and drug addiction (Miller, 1986; Miller & Hester, 1995). The result is one against which Jellinek warned: overlooking the important environmental determinants of substance-use disorders. The vast majority of addiction treatment continues to happen with only the client present (in individual or group sessions), searching within for the causes of the client's problems. It is abundantly clear that context is important in the etiology and maintenance of alcohol and other drug dependence. Relapse upon discharge to the natural environment is a classic problem in inpatient and residential treatment, which usually represent the most extreme end of the "fix the person" continuum. When the problem is seen as lying within the person, there is little reason to attend to (let alone get involved with) the social environment. In fact, such factors may be dismissed as "excuses". It is perhaps no coincidence, then, that CRA seems to have been more readily embraced in Scandinavian and other cultures where it is normative to conceptualize personal behavior and problems in their social context.

If I had a hammer

It really is hard to teach an old dog new tricks. There is truth to the adage, "If the only tool you have is a hammer, you tend to treat everything as if it were a nail." Established patterns of thought and practice may require unlearning before innovations can be learned and applied. Like other human beings, therapists are reluctant to re-evaluate cherished assumptions and familiar practices (Rogers, 1995). Doing CRA is hard work, and action-oriented. Learning CRA takes time and supervision.

Low excitement

CRA simply isn't sexy. It has no elaborate intrapsychic theory. When done well, there are usually no power struggles, no confrontation, no tearful and dramatic breakthroughs. The therapist doesn't cure the patient, or take credit for progress. CRA has no steps or slogans to memorize. It has no charismatic gurus. Even the name is a bit unfortunate: the Community Reinforcement Approach. Is it social casework? Are we reinforcing cities? What is it?

We already do that

A month after one of us had given an hour-long presentation on treatment methods that are supported by outcome studies, a local hospital released new advertising brochures claiming that their program used CRA (and just about everything else on our list of empirically supported methods). No one from the program had received any training in CRA. How does this happen? How do people becomes experts overnight and without any formal training?

A brief reading or hearing of CRA can lead to the quick conclusion that "we already do that". After all, isn't it just common sense that positive reinforcement is important, and that clients need to develop a new life-style? Yes, thankfully, it is. Yet good sense isn't always that common, at least in its application. When we observe tapes of therapists who believe that they are "doing CRA" (including our own trainees), we sometimes recognize little of what is being delivered. CRA is a systematic approach, not merely an idea or a few techniques.

What distinguishes CRA from other approaches?

This leads to another question that has challenged us over the years. What are the necessary and sufficient conditions of CRA? What is it that distinguishes this therapeutic approach from others? In particular, isn't this "just cognitive-behavioral therapy?"

Yes and no. To be sure, CRA arose from the empirical and theoretical traditions that gave rise to behavior therapy. Azrin was among the earliest and most innovative psychologists to apply learning theory and behavioral science to the resolution of serious clinical problems. CRA's cornerstone is positive reinforcement, basic B.F. Skinner. It is a fundamentally contextual way of thinking about and addressing behavior problems. It relies upon a careful individual functional analysis of behavior. CRA has all of that in common historically with behavior therapy.

Ironically, it is precisely at those points where CRA, in our view, differs from much of modern cognitive-behavior therapy. At the risk of sounding like back-to-basics fundamentalists, we find that many behavior therapists pay surprisingly little attention to social reinforcement contingencies. Functional analysis, if done at all, is often informal and perfunctory. Gathering data about behavioral contingencies in the natural environment has become a rare event. For better or worse, large amounts of attention are devoted to cognitions and beliefs that reside within the individual client. If there is a general theory that characterizes American behavior therapy at present, it is not classic or operant learning, but rather the idea that people get into trouble because they are deficient in coping skills. Identify the self-management deficit that underlies the problem, pull the appropriate skill-training approach off the shelf, and start teaching the right cognitive-behavioral coping procedures.

We quickly acknowledge that there is merit to therapies based on a skill-training model. Pragmatic empiricism does continue to characterize cognitive-behavioral approaches. Outcome research supports the efficacy of cognitive therapy for depression, and of social skills training for alcohol problems. While we are not persuaded that skill acquisition is the actual mechanism by which these therapies operate, something is working. Indeed, CRA includes behavior rehearsal and reinforcement of successive approximations.

In many ways, CRA *is* good behavior therapy. The difference we see is one of systematic emphasis. The three most important components of CRA are reinforcement, reinforcement, and reinforcement. How can one reinforce the person within sessions to come to and participate in treatment? What is reinforcing the person's current ("problem") behavior? What reinforcers could override the status quo, to establish a new and stable behavior pattern? The CRA therapist's eye is always on the reinforcers. Little emphasis is given to cognitions. Significant others are involved in treatment, and are taught how to make use of reinforcement contingencies in behavior change. Brief behavioral coaching may be used to help a client deal with a specific obstacle or initiate a new pattern of behavior that can be maintained by natural positive reinforcement. Very practical assistance is provided to boost the client's naturally occurring level of positive reinforcement for problem-inconsistent behavior. The menu of procedures is a tool box to be used creatively toward the ever-visible single-minded goal of enhancing positive reinforcement for new nondestructive behavior patterns. None of this is strange to behavior therapists; it is a matter of systematic focus and emphasis.

Future directions

Diffusion

Where will CRA go from here? Like a number of other methods, it is a treatment approach with solid evidence of efficacy, awaiting transfer to clinical practice. Additional clinical trials demonstrating its efficacy with substance-use disorders are unlikely to trigger its adoption into treatment systems. The next step, then, is to facilitate (and study) the dissemination of CRA into routine practice. What does it take for novice or experienced clinicians to learn this approach, and be able to deliver it as a systematic treatment? How well is the approach maintained over the months or years of practice after initial training? The leap from efficacy (clinical trials) to effectiveness (real-life treatment systems) is not a long one, in part because most of the studies reported in this book were done in the context of ongoing substance-abuse treatment programs. Yet, are the outcomes as good when CRA is learned and applied in clinical programs, outside the context of outcome research? What factors determine whether clinicians learn and maintain CRA practices, and, when they do, are the outcomes for their clients improved?

Generalization

Beyond diffusion efforts, another future direction for CRA is its application to other clinical problems. There is nothing about CRA that is specific to addictive behaviors. It is a general positive reinforcement approach that could be applied to increase or decrease a wide range of health-related behaviors. CRA procedures that have been applied effectively to increase disulfiram compliance could also be used to promote adherence to other pharmacotherapies. Reinforcement-based treatment procedures have been effective in managing pain, depression, and marital/family distress. They might be applied to enhance adherence to diabetes management, cardiovascular rehabilitation, physical therapy and exercise, and weight management programs. Indeed, CRA was just one of Azrin's many creative applications of operant psychology to the treatment of vexing clinical problems.

Service delivery

Large geographical areas have no mental health services within easy reach. Many who do have access are reluctant, afraid, embarrassed, or otherwise unwilling to seek such services in person. If CRA can be delivered effectively in person, most likely there are other formats in which it could be delivered as well: by telephone, by computer, perhaps even in printed form or by mail. How could CRA be made available to a larger population through media such as these, and how effective would it be relative to in-person treatment?

Other populations

It also seems feasible to apply CRA to other settings. We are studying CRA and CRAFT treatment for troubled adolescents and their families. How might this systematic positive social reinforcement approach be applied to address problems in nursing homes, in correctional settings, in public welfare systems, and in schools?

In short, CRA is not merely a set of techniques, but a general philosophy and approach that may have many cost-effective applications. The practical approach has been well specified, and its efficacy in treating substance-use disorders has been carefully documented in clinical trials spanning 30 years. It remains to be seen whether this large body of work will eventually find its way into effective practice, or be quietly archived on the bookshelves of history.

References

Abbott, P. J., Moore, B. A., Weller, A. B. & Delaney, H. D. (1998*a*). AIDS risk behaviors in opioid dependent patients treated with Community Reinforcement Approach and relationships with psychiatric disorders. *Journal of Addictive Diseases*, **17**, 33–48.

Abbott, P. J., Weller, S. B., Delaney, H. D. & Moore, B. A. (1998*b*). Community Reinforcement Approach in the treatment of opiate addicts. *American Journal of Drug and Alcohol Abuse*, **24**, 17–30.

American Psychiatric Association (1980). *Diagnostic and statistical manual of mental disorders* (3rd edn.). Washington, DC: American Psychiatric Association.

American Psychiatric Association (1987). *Diagnostic and statistical manual of mental disorders* (3rd edn., revised). Washington, DC: American Psychiatric Association.

Argeriou, M., McCarty, D., Mulvey, K. & Daley, M. (1994). Use of the Addiction Severity Index with homeless substance abusers. *Journal of Substance Abuse Treatment*, **11**, 359–365.

Armor, D. J., Polich, J. M., Stambul, H. B. (1976). *Alcoholism and treatment*. Santa Monica, CA: Rand Corporation.

Attkisson, C. C. & Zwick, R. (1982). The Client Satisfaction Questionnaire: psychometric properties and correlations with service utilization and psychotherapy outcome. *Evaluation & Program Planning*, **5**, 233–237.

Azrin, N. (1976). Improvements in the community-reinforcement approach to alcoholism. *Behaviour Research and Therapy*, **14**, 339–348.

Azrin, N., Acierno, R., Kogan, E. S., Donohue, B., Besalel, V. A. & McMahon, P. T. (1996). Follow-up results of supportive versus behavioral therapy for illicit drug use. *Behaviour Research and Therapy*, **34**, 41–46.

Azrin, N. & Besalel, V. A. (1980). *Job club counselor's manual*. Baltimore, MD: University Press.

Azrin, N. & Besalel, V. A. (1982). *Finding a job*. Berkeley, CA: Ten Speed Press.

Azrin, N., Besalel, V. A., Bechtel, R., Michalicek, A., Mancera, M., Carroll, D., Shuford, D. & Cox, J. (1980). Comparison of reciprocity and discussion-type counseling for marital problems. *American Journal of Family Therapy*, **8**, 21–28.

Azrin, N., Donohue, B. C., Besalel, V. A., Acierno, R. & Kogan, E. S. (1994). A new role for psychology in the treatment of drug abuse. *Psychotherapy in Private Practice*, **13**, 73–80.

Azrin, N., Flores, R. & Kaplan, S. J. (1975). Job-finding club: A group-assisted program for obtaining employment. *Behaviour Research and Therapy*, **13**, 17–24.

Azrin, N. H. & Fox, R. M. (1976). *Toilet training in less than a day*. New York: Simon & Schuster.

Azrin, N., Naster, B. J. & Jones, R. (1973). Reciprocity counseling: a rapid learning-based procedure for marital counseling. *Behaviour Research and Therapy*, **11**, 365–382.

Azrin, N., Nunn, R. G. & Frantz, S. E. (1980). Habit reversal vs. negative practice treatment of nervous tics. *Behavior Therapy*, **11**, 169–178.

Azrin, N., Philip, R. A., Thienes-Hontos, P. & Besalel, V. A. (1981). Follow-up on welfare benefits received by Job Club clients. *Journal of Vocational Behavior*, **18**, 253–254.

Azrin, N., Sisson, R. W., Meyers, R. J. & Godley, M. (1982). Alcoholism treatment by disulfiram and community reinforcement therapy. *Journal of Behavior Therapy and Experimental Psychiatry*, **13**, 105–112.

Baekeland, F. & Lundwall, L. (1975). Dropping out of treatment: a critical review. *Psychological Bulletin*, **82**, 738–783.

Ball, J. C. & Ross, A. (1991). *The effectiveness of methadone maintenance treatment*. New York: Springer-Verlag.

Beck, A. T., Ward, C. H., Mendelson, M., Mock, J. & Erbaugh, J. (1961). An inventory for measuring depression. *Archives of General Psychiatry*, **4**, 561–571.

Besalel, V. A. & Azrin, N. H. (1981). The reduction of parent–youth problems by reciprocity counseling. *Behaviour Research and Therapy*, **19**, 297–301.

Bickel, W. K. & Amass, L. (1995). Buprenorphine treatment of opioid dependence: a review. *Experimental and Clinical Psychopharmacology*, **3**, 477–489.

Bickel, W. K., Amass, L., Higgins, S. T., Badger, G. J. & Esch, R. A. (1997). Effects of adding behavioral treatment to opioid detoxification with buprenorphine. *Journal of Consulting and Clinical Psychology*, **65**, 803–810.

Bickel, W. K., Stitzer, M. L., Bigelow, G. E., Liebson, I. A., Jasinski, D. R. & Johnson, R. E. (1988). A clinical trial of buprenorphine: comparison with methadone in the detoxification of heroin addicts. *Clinical Pharmacology and Therapeutics*, **43**, 72–78.

Bonham, G. S., Hague, D. E., Abel, M. H., Cummings, P. & Deutsch, R. S. (1990). Louisville's Project Connect for the homeless alcohol and drug abuser. *Alcoholism Treatment Quarterly*, **7**, 57–78.

Braucht, G. N., Reichardt, C. S., Geissler, L. J., Bormann, C. A., Kwiatkowski, C. F. & Kirby, M. W. (1995). Effective services for homeless substance abusers. *Journal of Addictive Diseases*, **14**, 87–109.

Brewington, V., Arella, L., Deren, S. & Randell, J. (1987). Obstacles to the utilization of vocational services: an analysis of the literature. *The International Journal of the Addictions*, **22**, 1091–1118.

Brickman, P., Rabinowitz, V. C. & Karuza, J. (1982). Models of helping and coping. *American Psychologist*, **37**, 368–384.

Brown, T. G., Kokin, M., Seraganian, P. & Shields, N. (1995). The role of spouses of substance abusers in treatment: gender differences. *Journal of Psychoactive Drugs*, **27**, 223–229.

Budney, A. J. & Higgins, S. T. (1998). *National Institute on Drug Abuse therapy manuals for drug addiction: Manual 2. A Community Reinforcement Approach: treating cocaine addiction.* (NIH Publication No. 98–4309). Rockville, MD: U.S. Department of Health and Human Services.

Budney, A. J., Higgins, S. T., Delaney, D. D., Kent, L. & Bickel, W. K. (1991). Contingent reinforcement of abstinence with individuals abusing cocaine and marijuana. *Journal of Applied Behavior Analysis*, **24**, 657–665.

Carroll, K. M. (1999). Behavioral and cognitive behavioral treatments. In: B. S. McCrady & E. E. Epstein (eds.) *Addictions: a comprehensive guidebook* (pp. 250–267). New York: Oxford University Press.

Carroll, K. M., Nich, C., Ball, S. A., McCance, E. & Rounsaville, B. J. (1998). Treatment of cocaine and alcohol dependence with psychotherapy and disulfiram. *Addiction*, **93**, 713–728.

Carroll, K. M., Ziedonis, D., O'Malley, S., McCance-Katz, E., Gordon, L. & Rounsaville, B. (1993). Pharmacologic interventions for alcohol- and cocaine-abusing individuals: a pilot study of disulfiram vs. naltrexone. *The American Journal on Addictions*, **2**, 77–79.

Caton, C. L., Wyatt, R. J., Felix, A., Grunberg, J. & Dominguez, B. (1993). Follow-up of chronically homeless mentally ill men. *American Journal of Psychiatry*, **150**, 1639–1642.

Coleman, D. H. & Straus, M. A. (1986). Marital power, conflict, and violence in a nationally representative sample of American couples. *Violence & Victims*, **1**, 141–157.

Collins, R. L., Leonard, K. E. & Searles, J. S. (eds.). (1990). *Alcohol and the family: research and clinical perspectives.* New York: Guilford Press.

Cowell, A. (1997). The opium kings (A. Cowell, Director). In: R. James (Executive Producer) *Frontline.* New York and Washington, DC: Public Broadcasting Service.

Davies D. L. (1962) Normal drinking in recovered alcohol addicts. *Quarterly Journal of Studies on Alcohol*, **23**, 94–104.

Derogatis, L. R. (1983) Misuse of the Symptom Checklist 90 [letter]. *Archives of General Psychiatry*, **40**, 1152–1153.

Derogatis, L. R. & Melisaratos, N. (1983). The Brief Symptom Inventory: an introductory report. *Psychological Medicine*, **13**, 595–605.

Derogatis, L. R., Rickels, K. & Rock, A. F. (1976). The SCL-90 and the MMPI: a step in the validation of a new self-report scale. *British Journal of Psychiatry*, **128**, 280–289.

DiClemente, C. C. & Hughes, S. O. (1990). Stages of change profiles in outpatient alcoholism treatment. *Journal of Substance Abuse*, **2**, 217–235.

Drake, R. E., McHugo, G. J. & Biesanz, J. C. (1995). The test–retest reliability of standardized instruments among homeless persons with substance use disorders. *Journal of Studies on Alcohol*, **56**, 161–167.

Drake, R. E. & Wallach, M. A. (1989). Substance abuse among the chronic mentally ill. *Hospital and Community Psychiatry*, **40**, 1041–1046.

Dreese, M. (1960). *How to get the job* (revised edition). Chicago, IL: Science Research Associates.

D'Zurilla, T. J. & Goldfried, M. R. (1971). Problem solving and behavior modification. *Journal of Abnormal Psychology*, **78**, 107–126.

Ellis, B. H., McCan, I., Price, G. & Sewell, C. M. (1992). The New Mexico Treatment Outcome Study: evaluating the utility of existing information systems. *Journal of Health Care for the Poor & Underserved*, **3**, 138–150.

Fals-Stewart, W., Birchler, G. R. & O'Farrell, T. J. (1996). Behavioral couples therapy for male substance abusing patients: effects on relationship adjustment and drug–using behavior. *Journal of Consulting and Clinical Psychology*, **64**, 959–972.

Finney, J. W. & Monahan, S. C. (1996). The cost-effectiveness of treatment for alcoholism: a second approximation. *Journal of Studies on Alcohol*, **57**, 229–243.

Fischer, P. J. (1988). Criminal activity among the homeless: a study of arrests in Baltimore. *Hospital & Community Psychiatry*, **39**, 46–51.

Fischer, P. J. (1989). Estimating prevalence of alcohol, drug, and mental health problems in the contemporary homeless population: a review of the literature. *Contemporary Drug Problems*, **16**, 333–390.

Fischer, P. J. & Breakey, W. R. (1991). The epidemiology of alcohol, drug, and mental disorders among homeless persons. *American Psychologist*, **46**, 1115–1128.

Foote, A., Googins, B., Moriarty, M., Sandonato, C., Nadolski, J. & Jefferson, C. (1994). Implementing long-term EAP follow-up with clients and family members to help prevent relapse with implications for primary prevention. *Journal of Primary Prevention*, **15**, 173–191.

Forgays, D. K., Spielberger, C. D., Ottaway, S. A. & Forgays, D. G. (1998). Factor structure of the State–Trait Anger Expression Inventory for middle-aged men and women. *Assessment*, **5**, 141–155.

Fox, R. (1967). Disulfiram (Antabuse) as an adjunct in the treatment of alcoholism. In: R. Fox (ed.) *Alcoholism: behavioral research, therapeutic approaches*. New York, NY: Springer-Verlag.

Geissler, L., Bormann, C., Kwiatowski, C., Braucht, G. & Reichardt, C. (1995). Women, homelessness, and substance abuse: moving beyond the stereotypes. *Psychology of Women Quarterly*, **19**, 65–83.

Gelberg, L., Linn, L. S. & Leake, B. D. (1988). Mental health, alcohol and drug use, and criminal history among homeless adults. *American Journal of Psychiatry*, **145**, 191–196.

Gondolf, E. W. & Foster, R. A. (1991). Wife assault among VA alcohol rehabilitation patients. *Hospital & Community Psychiatry*, **42**, 74–79.

Grant, K. A., Arciniega, L. M., Tonigan, J. S., Miller, W. R. & Meyers, R. J. (1997). Are reconstructed self-reports of drinking reliable? *Addiction*, **92**, 601–606.

Grella, C. E. (1993). A residential recovery program for homeless alcoholics: differences in program recruitment and retention. *The Journal of Mental Health Administration*, **20**, 90–99.

Griffiths, R. R., Bigelow, G. E. & Henningfield, J. E. (1980). Similarities in animal and human drug taking behavior. In: N. K. Mellow (ed.) *Advances in substance abuse: behavioral and biological research* (pp. 1–90). Greenwich, CT: JAI Press.

Griffiths, R. R., Bigelow, G. E. & Liebson, I. A. (1978). Relationship of social factors to ethanol self-administration in alcoholics. In: P. E. Nathan, G. A. Marlatt & T. T. Loberg (eds.) *New directions in behavioral research and treatment* (pp. 351–379). New York: Plenum Press.

Hamilton, M. (1960). A rating scale for depression. *Journal of Neurology, Neurosurgery, and Psychiatry*, **23**, 56–61.

Harris, R. (1985). *A primer of multivariate statistics*. Orlando, FL: Academic Press.

Heather, N. & Robertson, I. (1962). *Controlled drinking*. London: Methuen.

Hedges, L. V. & Olkin, I. (1985). *Statistical methods for meta-analysis*. Orlando, FL: Academic Press.

Higgins, S. T., Badger, G. J. & Budney, A. J. (2000). Duration of initial cocaine abstinence and success in achieving longer-term abstinence. (in press)

Higgins, S. T. & Budney, A. J. (1997). From the initial clinic contact to aftercare: a brief review of effective strategies for retaining cocaine abusers in treatment. In: L. S. Onken, J. D. Blaine & J. J. Boren (eds.) *Beyond the therapeutic alliance: keeping the drug-dependent individual in treatment.* National Institute on Drug Abuse Monograph Series, no. 165 (pp. 25–43). NIH publication No. 97–4142. Washington, DC: Supt. of Docs., U.S. Government Printing Office.

Higgins, S. T., Budney, A. J., Bickel, W. K. & Badger, G. J. (1994a). Participation of significant others in outpatient behavioral treatment predicts greater cocaine abstinence. *American Journal of Drug and Alcohol Abuse*, **20**, 47–56.

Higgins, S. T., Budney, A. J., Bickel, W. K., Foerg, F. E. & Badger, G. J. (1994b). Alcohol dependence and simultaneous cocaine and alcohol use in cocaine-dependent patients. *Journal of Addictive Diseases*, **13**, 177–189.

Higgins, S. T., Budney, A. J., Bickel, W. K., Foerg, F. E., Donham, R. & Badger, G. J. (1994c). Incentives improve treatment retention and cocaine abstinence in ambulatory cocaine-dependent patients. *Archives of General Psychiatry*, **51**, 568–576.

Higgins, S. T., Budney, A. J., Bickel, W. K., Foerg, F. E., Ogden, D. & Badger, G. J. (1995). Outpatient behavioral treatment for cocaine dependence: one-year outcome. *Experimental and Clinical Psychopharmacology*, **3**, 205–212.

Higgins, S. T., Budney, A. J., Bickel, W. K., Hughes, J. R. & Foerg, F. (1993a). Disulfiram therapy in patients abusing cocaine and alcohol. *American Journal of Psychiatry*, **150**, 675–676.

Higgins, S. T., Budney, A. J., Bickel, W. K., Hughes, J. R., Foerg, F. & Badger, G. (1993b). Achieving cocaine abstinence with a behavioral approach. *American Journal of Psychiatry*, **150**, 763–769.

Higgins, S. T., Delaney, D. D., Budney, A. J., Bickel, W. K., Hughes, J. R., Foerg, F. & Fenwick, J. W. (1991). A behavioral approach to achieving initial cocaine abstinence. *American Journal of Psychiatry*, **148**, 1218–1224.

Higgins, S. T. & Silverman, K. (eds.) (1999). *Motivating behavior change among illicit-drug abusers: research on contingency management interventions.* Washington, DC: American Psychological Association.

Higgins, S. T. & Wong, C. J. (1998). Treating cocaine abuse: what does research tell us? In: S. T. Higgins & J. L. Katz (eds.) *Cocaine abuse: behavior, pharmacology, and clinical applications* (pp. 343–361). San Diego, CA: Academic Press.

Higgins, S. T., Wong, C. J., Badger, G. J., Haug Ogden, D. E. & Dantona, R. L. (2000). Contingent reinforcement increases cocaine abstinence during outpatient treatment and one year of follow-up. *Journal of Consulting and Clinical Psychology*, **68**, 64–72.

Holder, H., Longabaugh, R., Miller, W. R. & Rubonis, A. (1991). The cost effectiveness of treatment for alcoholism: a first approximation. *Journal of Studies on Alcohol*, **52**, 517–540.

Holmberg, S. (1996). The estimated prevalence and incidence of HIV in 96 large US metropolitan areas. *The American Journal of Public Health*, **86**, 642–654.

Horn, J. L., Wanberg, K. & Foster, F. M. (1987). *The alcohol use inventory (revised)*. Minneapolis, MN: National Computer Systems.

Hunt, G. M. & Azrin, N. H. (1973). A community-reinforcement approach to alcoholism. *Behaviour Research and Therapy*, **11**, 91–104.

Institute of Medicine. (1988). *Homelessness, health, and human needs.* Washington, DC: National Academy Press.

Jellinek, E. M. (1960). *The disease concept of alcoholism.* New Haven, CT: College and University Press.

Jellinek, E. M. & Keller, M. (1952). Rates of alcoholism in the United States of America, 1940–1948. *Quarterly Journal of Studies on Alcohol*, **13**, 49–59.

Joe, G. W., Chastain, R. L. & Simpson, D. W. (1990). Relapse. In: D. D. Simpson & S. B. Sells (eds.) *Opioid addiction and treatment: a 12-year follow-up* (pp. 121–136). Malabar, FL: Krieger.

Johnston, L. D., O'Malley, P. M. & Bachman, J. G. (1997). *National survey results on drug use from the Monitoring the Future Study, 1975–1995: college students and young adults (Volume II)*. Rockville MD: National Institute on Drug Abuse.

Jones, R. J. & Azrin, N. H. (1973). An experimental application of a social reinforcement approach to the problem of job-finding. *Journal of Applied Behavioral Analysis*, **6**, 345–353.

Kogan, K. L. & Jacobson, J. (1965). Stress, personality and emotional disturbance in wives of alcoholics. *Quarterly Journal of Studies on Alcohol*, **26**, 486–495.

Konkol, R. J. & Olsen, G. D. (eds.) (1996). *Prenatal cocaine exposure.* New York: CRC Press.

Kraml, M. (1973). Letter: a rapid test for Antabuse ingestion. *Journal of the Canadian Medical Association*, **109**, 578.

Kristenson, H., Ohlin, H., Hulten-Nosslin, M. B. & Trell, E. (1983). Identification and intervention of heavy drinking in middle-aged men: results and follow-up of 24–60 months of long-term study with randomized controls. *Alcoholism: Clinical & Experimental Research*, **7**, 203–209.

Lapham, S. C., Hall, M. & Skipper, B. J. (1995). Homelessness and substance use among alcohol abusers following participation in Project HEART. *Journal of Addictive Diseases*, **14**, 41–55.

Leonard, K. E. & Jacob, T. (1988). Alcohol, alcoholism, and family violence. In: V. B. Van Hasselt, R. L. Morrison, A. S. Belleck & M. Hersen. (eds.) *Handbook of family violence* (pp. 383–406). New York: Plenum Press.

Lovibond, S. H. & Caddy, G. (1970). Discriminated averse control in the moderation of alcoholics' drinking behavior. *Behavior Therapy*, **1**, 437–444.

Lundwall, L. & Baekeland, F. (1971). Disulfiram treatment of alcoholism: a review. *Journal of Nervous and Mental Disorders*, **153**, 381–394.

Mallams, J. H., Godley, M. D., Hall, G. M. & Meyers, R. J. (1982). A social-systems approach to resocializing alcoholics in the community. *Journal of Studies on Alcohol*, **43**, 1115–1123.

Manson, M. P. & Lerner, A. (1962). *The Marriage Adjustment Inventory*. Los Angeles, CA: Western Psychological Services.

Markham, M. R., Miller, W. R. & Arciniega, L. (1993). BACCuS 2.01: computer software for quantifying alcohol consumption. *Behavior Research Methods, Instruments, and Computers*, **25**, 420–421.

Marlatt, G. A. & Gordon, J. R. (eds.). (1985). *Relapse prevention: maintenance strategies in the treatment of addictive behaviors.* New York, NY: Guilford Press.

McCarty, A. T., Argeriou, M., Huebner, R. & Lubran, B. (1991). Alcoholism, drug abuse and the homeless. *American Psychologist*, **46**, 1139–1148.

McCarty, A. T., Argeriou, M., Krakow, M. & Mulvey, K. (1990). Stabilization services for homeless alcoholics and drug addicts. *Alcoholism Treatment Quarterly*, **7**, 31–45.

McLellan, A. T., Arndt, I. O., Metzger, D. S., Woody, G. E. & O'Brien, C. P. (1993). The effects of psychosocial services in substance abuse treatment. *JAMA*, **269**, 1953–1959.

McLellan, A. T., Luborsky, L. & Cacciola, J. (1985). New data from the Addiction Severity Index: reliability and validity in three centers. *Journal of Nervous and Mental Diseases*, **173**, 412–423.

McLellan, A. T., Luborsky, L., O'Brien, C. P. & Woody, G. E. (1980). An improved diagnostic evaluation instrument for substance abuse patients: the Addiction Severity Index. *Journal of Nervous and Mental Disease*, **168**, 26–33.

Mendelson, J. H. & Mello, N. K. (1996). Management of cocaine abuse and dependence. *The New England Journal of Medicine*, **334**, 965–972.

Meyers, R. J., Dominguez, T. & Smith, J. E. (1996). Community reinforcement training with concerned others. In: V. B. Hasselt & M. Hersen (eds.) *Source of psychological treatment manuals for adult disorders* (pp. 257–294). New York, NY: Plenum Press.

Meyers, R. J., Miller, W. R., Hill, D. E. & Tonigan, J. S. (1999). Community reinforcement and family training (CRAFT): engaging unmotivated drug users in treatment. *Journal of Substance Abuse*, **10**, 291–308.

Meyers, R. J. & Smith, J. E. (1995). *Clinical guide to alcohol treatment: the Community Reinforcement Approach.* New York, NY: Guilford Press.

Meyers, R. J. & Smith, J. E. (1997). Getting off the fence: procedures to engage treatment-resistant drinkers. *Journal of Substance Abuse Treatment*, **14**, 467–472.

Meyers, R. J., Smith, J. E. & Miller, E. J. (1998). Working through the concerned significant other. In: W. R. Miller & N. Heather (eds.) *Treating addictive behaviors* (2nd edn.) (pp. 149–161). New York, NY: Plenum Press.

Meyers, R. J. & Wolfe, B. L. (1998). Community reinforcement and family training for families of substance abusers. *The Counselor*, November/December, 24–29.

Miller, W. R. (1986). Haunted by the *Zeitgeist*: reflections on contrasting treatment goals and concepts of alcoholism in Europe and the United States. *Annals of the New York Academy of Sciences*, **472**, 110–129.

Miller, W. R. (1996). What is a relapse? Fifty ways to leave the wagon. *Addiction*, **91** (Supplement), S15–S27.

Miller, W. R., Brown, J. M., Simpson, T. L., Handmaker, N. S., Bien, T. H., Luckie, L. F., Montgomery, H. A., Hester, R. K. & Tonigan, J. S. (1995). What works? A methodological analysis of the alcohol treatment outcome literature. In: R. K. Hester & W. R. Miller (eds.) *Handbook of alcoholism treatment approaches: effective alternatives* (2nd edn.) (pp. 12–44). Boston, MA: Allyn and Bacon.

Miller, W. R., Crawford, V. L. & Taylor, C. A. (1979). Significant others as corroborative sources for problem drinkers. *Addictive Behaviors*, **4**, 67–70.

Miller, W. R., Heather, N. & Hall, W. (1991). Calculating standard drink units: international comparisons. *British Journal of Addiction*, **86**, 43–47.

Miller, W. R. & Hester, R. K. (1986). The effectiveness of alcoholism treatment: what research reveals. In: W. R. Miller & N. Heather (eds.) *Treating addictive behaviors: processes of change* (pp. 121–174). New York, NY: Plenum Press.

Miller, W. R. & Hester, R. K. (1995). Treatment for alcohol problems: toward an informed eclecticism. In: R. K. Hester & W. R. Miller (eds.) *Handbook of alcoholism treatment approaches: effective alternatives* (2nd edn.) (pp. 1–11). Boston, MA: Allyn and Bacon.

Miller, W. R. & Marlatt, G. A. (1984). *Manual for the Comprehensive Drinker Profile*. Odessa, FL: Psychological Assessment Resources.

Miller, W. R. & Marlatt, G. A. (1987). *Manual for the Brief Drinker Profile*. Odessa, FL: Psychological Assessment Resources.

Miller, W. R., Meyers, R. J. & Hiller-Sturmhöfel, S. (1999). The community-reinforcement approach. *Alcohol Health & Research World*, **22**, 116–121.

Miller, W. R., Meyers, R. J. & Tonigan, J. S. (1999). Engaging the unmotivated in treatment for alcohol problems: a comparison of three strategies for intervention through family members. *Journal of Consulting and Clinical Psychology*, **67**, 688–697.

Miller, W. R. & Page, A. C. (1991). Warm turkey: other routes to abstinence. *Journal of Substance Abuse Treatment*, **8**, 227–232.

Miller, W. R. & Tonigan, J. S. (1996). Assessing drinkers' motivations for change: the Stages of Change Readiness and Treatment Eagerness Scale (SOCRATES). *Psychology of Addictive Behaviors*, **10**, 81–89.

Montoya, I. D. & Atkinson, J. S. (1996). Determinants of HIV seroprevalence rates among sites participating in a community based study of drug use. *Journal of Acquired Immune Deficiency Syndromes and Human Retrovirology*, **13**, 169–176.

Moos, R. & Moos, B. (1986). *Family environment scale manual*. Palo Alto, CA: Consulting Psychologists Press.

Moos, R. H., Finney, J. W. & Gamble, W. (1982). The process of recovery from alcoholism: II. Comparing spouses of alcoholic patients and matched community controls. *Journal of Studies on Alcohol*, **43**, 888–909.

Najavits, L. M. & Weiss, R. D. (1994). Variations in therapist effectiveness in the treatment of patients with substance use disorders: an empirical review. *Addiction*, **89**, 679–688.

National Institute of Justice. (1999). *1998 Annual report on cocaine use among arrestees, National Institute of Justice Research Report, 1999.* Rockville, MD: National Institute of Justice Clearinghouse.

National Institute on Alcohol Abuse and Alcoholism. (1991). *Alcohol, drug abuse and mental health problems among homeless persons: a review of the literature, 1980–1990* (DHHS Publication No. ADM 91–1763). Rockville, MD: U. S. Government Printing Office.

National Institute on Alcohol Abuse and Alcoholism. (1992*a*). *Homeless families with children: research perspectives.* (DHHS Publication No. ADM 92–1848). Rockville, MD: U.S. Government Printing Office.

National Institute on Alcohol Abuse and Alcoholism. (1992*b*). *Community demonstration grant projects for alcohol and drug abuse treatment of homeless individuals.* (NIH Publication No. 93–3537). Rockville, MD: Government Printing Office.

NIDA Notes. (1998). Volume 13, Number 2. Rockville, MD: National Clearinghouse for Alcohol and Drug Information.

Onken, L. S., Blaine, J. D. & Boren, J. J. (eds.) (1995). *Integrating behavioral therapies with medications in the treatment of drug dependence. National Institute on Drug Abuse Monograph Series, # 150.* (NIH publication No. 95–3899). Washington, DC: Supt. of Docs., U.S. Government Printing Office.

Orford, J. & Harwin, J. (eds.) (1982). *Alcohol and the family.* London: Croom Helm.

Paolino, T. J. & McCrady, B. S. (1977). The alcoholic marriage: alternative perspectives. New York, NY: Grune & Stratton.

Platt, J. J. (1995). Vocational rehabilitation of drug abusers. *Psychological Bulletin*, **117**, 416–433.

Project MATCH Research Group. (1997). Matching alcoholism treatments to client heterogeneity: Project MATCH posttreatment drinking outcomes. *Journal of Studies on Alcohol*, **58**, 7–29.

Project MATCH Research Group (1998). Therapist effects in three treatments for alcohol problems. *Psychotherapy Research*, **8**, 455–474.

Rawson, R.A., McCann, M., Huber, A. & Shoptaw, S. (1999). Contingency management and relapse prevention as stimulant abuse treatment interventions. In: S. T. Higgins & K. Silverman (eds.) *Motivating behavior change among illicit-drug abusers: research on contingency management interventions* (pp. 57–74). Washington, DC: American Psychological Association.

Reyes, E. & Miller, W. R. (1980). Serum gamma-glutamyl transpeptidase as a diagnostic aid in problem drinkers. *Addictive Behaviors*, **5**, 59–65.

Rogers, E. M. (1995). *Diffusion of innovations* (4th edn.). New York, NY: Free Press.

Rosen, G. (1977). *The relaxation book: an illustrated self-help program.* Englewood Cliff, NJ: Prentice-Hall.

Rossi, P. H. (1990). The old homeless and the new homeless in historical perspective. *American Psychologist*, **45**, 954–959.

Rychtarik, R. G., Smith, P. O., Jones, S. L., Doerfler, L., Hale, R. & Prue, D. M. (1983). Assessing disulfiram compliance: validational study of an abbreviated breath test procedure. *Addictive Behaviors*, **8**, 361–368.

Schottenfeld, R. S., Pascale, R. & Sokolowski, S. (1992). Matching services to needs: vocational services for substance abusers. *Journal of Substance Abuse Treatment*, **9**, 3–8.

Selzer, M. L. (1971). The Michigan Alcoholism Screening Test: the quest for a new diagnostic instrument. *American Journal of Psychiatry*, **127**, 1653–1658.

Silverman, K., Higgins, S. T., Brooner, R. K., Montoya, I. D., Cone, E. J., Schuster, C. R. & Preston, K. L. (1996*a*). Sustained cocaine abstinence in methadone maintenance patients through voucher-based reinforcement therapy. *Archives of General Psychiatry*, **53**, 409–415.

Silverman, K., Wong, C. J., Higgins, S. T., Brooner, R. K., Montoya, I. D., Contoreggi, C., Umbricht-Schneiter, A., Schuster, C. R. & Preston, K. L. (1996*b*). Increasing opiate abstinence through voucher-based reinforcement therapy. *Drug and Alcohol Dependence*, **41**, 157–165.

Silverman, K., Wong, C. J., Umbricht-Schneiter, A., Montoya, I. D., Schuster, C. R. & Preston, K. L. (1998). Broad beneficial effects of cocaine abstinence reinforcement among methadone patients. *Journal of Consulting and Clinical Psychology*, **66**, 811–824.

Sisson, R. W. & Azrin, N. H. (1986). Family-member involvement to initiate and promote treatment of problem drinkers. *Journal of Behavior Therapy and Experimental Psychiatry*, **17**, 15–21.

Sisson, R. W. & Mallams, J. H. (1981). The use of systematic encouragement and community access procedures to increase attendance at Alcoholics Anonymous and Al-Anon meetings. *American Journal of Drug and Alcohol Abuse*, **8**, 371–376.

Skinner, B. F. (1938). *The behavior of organisms*. New York, NY: Appleton-Century-Crofts.

Smith, J. E. & Meyers, R. J. (1995). The community reinforcement approach. In: R. K. Hester & W. R. Miller (eds.) *Handbook of alcoholism treatment approaches: effective alternatives* (2nd edn.) (pp. 251–266). Boston, MA: Allyn and Bacon.

Smith, J. E., Meyers, R. J. & Delaney, H. D. (1998). The Community Reinforcement Approach with homeless alcohol-dependent individuals. *Journal of Consulting and Clinical Psychology*, **66**, 541–548.

Smith, J. E., Meyers, R. J. & Waldorf, V. A. (1999). Covering all bases: engaging and treating individuals with alcohol problems. In: J. H. Hannigan, L. P. Spear, N. E. Spear & C. R. Goodlett (eds.) *Alcohol and alcoholism: effects on brain and development* (pp. 229–249). Mahwah, NJ: Lawrence Erlbaum Associates, Inc.

Sobell, L. C. & Sobell, M. B. (1973*a*). A self-feedback technique to monitor drinking behavior in alcoholics. *Behaviour Research & Therapy*, **11**, 237–238.

Sobell, M. B. & Sobell, L. C. (1973*b*). Individualized behavior therapy for alcoholics. *Behavior Therapy*, **4**, 49–72.

Sobell, M. B. & Sobell, L. C. (1984). The aftermath of heresy: a response to Pendery et al.'s critique of "individualized behavior therapy for alcoholics." *Behaviour Research and Therapy*, **22**, 413–440.

Sosin, M. R., Bruni, M. & Reidy, M. (1995). Paths and impacts in the progressive independence model: A homelessness and substance abuse intervention in Chicago. *Journal of Addictive Diseases*, **14**, 1–20.

Sosin, M. R. & Yamaguchi, J. (1995). Case management routines and discretion in a program addressing homelessness and substance abuse. *Contemporary Drug Problems*, **22**, 317–342.

Spielberger, C. D. (1996). *State-Trait Anger Expression Inventory: professional manual*. (Revised research edition). Odessa, FL: Psychological Assessment Resources.

Spitzer, R. L., Williams, J. B. W., Gibbon, M. & First, M. B. (1988). *Structured clinical interview for DSM-III-R, patient version (SCID-P)*. New York, NY: Biometrics Research Department, New York State Psychiatric Institute.

Stitzer, M., Bickel, W. K., Bigelow, G. & Liebson, I. (1986). Effects of methadone dose contingencies on urinalysis test results of poly-abusing methadone-maintenance patients. *Drug and Alcohol Dependence*, **18**, 341–348.

Stahler, G. J. (1995). Social interventions for homeless substance abusers: evaluation treatment outcomes. *Journal of Addictive Diseases*, **14**, xv–xxvi.

Stambul, H. B. & Polich, J. M. (1977). *Some implications of the Rand Alcoholism and Treatment study for alcoholism research*. Santa Monica, CA: Rand Corporation.

Stark, M. J. & Campbell, B. K. (1988). Personality, drug use, and early attrition from substance abuse treatment. *American Journal of Drug & Alcohol Abuse*, **14**, 475–485.

Stine, S. M. & Kosten, T. R. (eds.) (1997). *New treatments for opiate dependence*. New York, NY: Guilford Press.

Stith, S. M., Crossman, R. K. & Bischof, G. P. (1991). Alcoholism and marital violence: a comparative study of men in alcohol treatment programs and batterer treatment programs. *Alcoholism Treatment Quarterly*, **8**, 3–20.

Straus, M. A. (1979). Measuring intrafamily conflict and violence: the Conflict Tactics (CT) Scales. *Journal of Marriage & The Family*, **41**, 75–88.

Stuart, R. B. (1969). Operant-interpersonal treatment for marital discord. *Journal of Consulting and Clinical Psychology*, **33**, 675–682.

Substance Abuse and Mental Health Services Administration. (SAMHSA) (1997*a*). *Preliminary results from the 1996 National Household Survey on Drug Abuse*. Rockville, MD: National Clearinghouse for Alcohol and Drug Information.

Substance Abuse and Mental Health Services Administration. (SAMHSA) (1997*b*). *National Household Survey on Drug Abuse: population estimates 1996*. Rockville, MD: National Clearinghouse for Alcohol and Drug Information.

Substance Abuse and Mental Heath Services Administration. (SAMHSA) (1997*c*). *Drug abuse warning network series: D-3: year-end preliminary estimates from the 1996 drug abuse warning network*. Rockville MD: National Clearinghouse for Alcohol and Drug Information.

Substance Abuse and Mental Health Services Administration. (SAMHSA) (1998). *National Household Survey on Drug Abuse: population estimates, 1997.* Rockville, MD: National Clearinghouse for Alcohol and Drug Information.

Tabachnick, B. & Fidell, L. (1989). *Using multivariate statistics.* New York, NY: Harper & Row.

Tardiff, K., Marzuk, P. M., Leon, A. C., Hirsch, C. S., Stajie, M., Portera, L. & Hartwell, N. (1994). Homicide in New York City: cocaine use and firearms. *Journal of the American Medical Association, 272,* 43–46.

Thomas, E. J. & Ager, R. D. (1993). Unilateral family therapy with spouses of uncooperative alcohol abusers. In: T. J. O'Farrell (ed.) *Treating alcohol problems: marital and family interventions* (pp. 3–33). New York, NY: Guilford Press.

Thomas, E. J., Yoshioka, M. & Ager, R. D. (1996). Spouse enabling of alcohol abuse: conception, assessment, and modification. *Journal of Substance Abuse, 8,* 61–80.

Toro, P. A., Passero Rabideau, J. M., Bellavia, C. W., Daeschler, C. V., Wall, D. D., Thomas, D. M. & Smith, S. J. (1997). Evaluating an intervention for homeless persons: results of a field experiment. *Journal of Consulting and Clinical Psychology, 65,* 476–484.

Velleman, R., Bennett, G., Miller, T., Orford, J., Rigby, K. & Tod, A. (1993). The families of problem drug users: a study of 50 close relatives. *Addiction, 88,* 1281–1289.

Welte, J. W. & Barnes, G. M. (1992). Drinking among homeless and marginally housed adults in New York State. *Journal of Studies on Alcohol, 53,* 303–315.

Willenbring, M. L., Whelen, J. A., Dahlquist, J. S. & O'Neal. M. E. (1990). Community treatment of the chronic public inebriate I: Implementation. *Alcoholism Treatment Quarterly, 7,* 79–98.

Wright, J. D. (1989). *Address unknown: the homeless in America.* New York, NY: Aldine de Gruyter.

Wright, J. D. & Weber, E. (1987). *Homeless & health.* New York, NY: McGraw-Hill.

Index